DRUG TESTING

DRUG TESTING:
Issues and Options

Edited by

Robert H. Coombs, Ph.D., and
Louis Jolyon West, M.D.
UCLA School of Medicine

New York   Oxford
Oxford University Press
1991

Oxford University Press

Oxford   New York   Toronto
Delhi   Bombay   Calcutta   Madras   Karachi
Petaling Jaya   Singapore   Hong Kong   Tokyo
Nairobi   Dar es Salaam   Cape Town
Melbourne   Auckland

and associated companies in
Berlin   Ibadan

Copyright © 1991 by Oxford University Press, Inc.

Published by Oxford University Press, Inc.
200 Madison Avenue, New York, New York 10016

Oxford is a registered trademark of Oxford University Press

Library of Congress Cataloging-in-Publication Data
Drug testing : issues and options
edited by R. H. Coombs and L. J. West.
p. cm.   Includes bibliographical references.   Includes index.
ISBN 0-19-505414-8
1. Drug testing—United States.
I. Coombs, Robert H.
II. West, Louis Jolyon, 1924–
[DNLM: 1. Civil Rights—United States.
2. Substance Abuse Detection.
WM 270 D7950034]
HV5823.5.U5D77   1991
362.29'364'0973—dc20   DLC
for Library of Congress   90-7848

9 8 7 6 5 4 3 2 1

Printed in the United States of America
on acid-free paper

For
Holly and Chip

ACKNOWLEDGMENTS

We acknowledge with appreciation the assistance of
Carla Cronkhite Vera, Deborah Ackerman,
Carol Jean Coombs, and Daniel Bloom.
Their participation greatly contributed to the
completion of this book.

Contents

Contributors

Deborah L. Ackerman, M.S. (pharmacology), is a research associate, UCLA School of Medicine and Ph.D. candidate, UCLA School of Public Health.

Robert T. Angarola, J.D., is an expert on food and drug law with the firm of Hyman, Phelps and McNamara, P.C., in Washington, D.C., and has testified before Congress on this topic.

Helen Axel, M.A., is a Senior Research Fellow at The Conference Board, a non-profit business and information service in New York.

Robert H. Coombs, Ph.D., is professor of biobehavioral sciences, UCLA School of Medicine, and director, Office of Education, UCLA Neuropsychiatric Institute and Hospital.

Bernard Lo, M.D., is associate professor of medicine, University of California-San Francisco, School of Medicine, and director of the Program in Medical Ethics, UCSF.

Paul J. Mulloy, Rear Admiral, U.S. Navy (Ret.) is president of P. J. Mulloy Associates, Inc., a private consulting firm in McLean, Virginia, and former head of the U.S. Navy's "War on Drugs."

Ronald M. Paolino, Ph.D., is clinical associate professor of psychiatry, Brown University Program in Medicine, former chief, Drug Dependency Treatment Program, VA Medical Center, Providence, Rhode Island, and president of a private consulting firm in Providence, Rhode Island.

Jeanne G. Trumble, M.S.W., is chief, Workplace Policy Research Branch in the Division of Applied Research of the National Institute on Drug Abuse.

J. Michael Walsh, Ph.D., is director, Division of Applied Research, National Institute on Drug Abuse.

Louis Jolyon West, M.D., is professor of Psychiatry, UCLA School of Medicine.

Robert E. Willette, Ph.D., is president of Duo Research, a private consulting firm in Annapolis, Maryland, and consultant, U.S. Navy.

Eric D. Zemper, Ph.D., is president of Exercise Research Associates of Oregon, a nonprofit research corporation in Eugene, Oregon.

Introduction

The evolving story of drug testing is complex, multifaceted, and controversial. Almost overnight, testing has grown into a $1 billion industry (Hafner & Garland, 1988). Amid national concern about illicit drug abuse, drug testing (mostly urinalysis) has burst upon the American scene as a contentious issue.

At work and at school, thousands of individuals are tested for drugs. Some acquiesce, others refuse; acrimonious conflicts and legal actions ensue. Despite abundant criticism, drug testing, called "the premier issue in labor relations for the next decade," has become an established part of American society (Kaufman, 1986).

Most Americans find it easy to be on both sides of the issue at once and to vacillate from one point of view to the other as each side argues its case. On the one hand, it is a relief to see something effective being done to curtail the ever-growing and worrisome problem of drug abuse. Yet drug testing is an invasion of privacy. "I have mixed feelings, I really do," a mother confessed. "I'm afraid for my son, but where do you stop? Next thing you know, we're going to be testing the preacher. I may end up being 49.5 percent in favor and 49.5 percent opposed" (Applebome, 1986).

Even among the most vocal combatants, the battle lines in this dispute are not always neatly drawn. Internal disagreements have arisen among some unions and employee groups, for example, whether to oppose or support drug testing. A drug-free, safe workplace is appealing to all employees, but mandatory testing can be a control issue, a humiliating intrusion by management into a subordinate's privacy. Neither are all employers singleminded about how strictly to enforce drug testing, who to test, and in what circumstances.

Those who favor drug testing, insisting that employers have the right to demand a drug-free work force, point to absenteeism, diminished productivity, increased accidents, medical claims, and theft as results of drug abuse. "Drug abuse is an economic hemorrhage on the business community," said an executive of the Institute for a Drug-Free Workplace. A Gallup Poll commissioned by the institute found one in four U.S. workers aware of co-workers who use illegal drugs on the job. Estimated losses resulting from drug abuse are $60 billion annually (Kelley, 1989).

Drug screening got its start in the 1960s amid reports that American soldiers in Vietnam were becoming addicted to heroin and other drugs. In the 1970s, the Department of Defense developed drug-detection programs to identify and treat returning heroin-addicted GIs. Today, each branch of the military services conducts drug testing.

In July 1986, President Ronald Reagan announced a plan to test government employees, extending the existing testing procedures of such agencies as the Federal Bureau of Investigation, the Immigration and Naturalization Service, the Federal Aviation Administration, the Postal Service, the Drug Enforcement Administration, and the military services. Urging that "voluntary" drug testing be considered both in and out of the government, he and Vice-President George Bush underwent urinalysis along with seventy-eight members of the senior White House staff. Two months later, President Reagan signed an Executive Order calling for drug testing on a broad range of the federal government's 2.8 million civilian employees. This decree earmarked $56 million for the first year of this undertaking. The rules, written by the government's Office of Personnel Management, stipulated that federal agency and government heads may fire workers in sensitive positions, such as those with access to classified information, who are found to use illegal drugs. Supervisors were to notify affected employees thirty days in advance that they are required to be tested. Those who refused risked being fired.

By the following year, the amount of drug testing is thought to have doubled (Lunzer, 1987). Testing spread not just in federal agencies but also in a growing number of local police and fire departments. The call has even gone out for the testing of judges and attorneys, and the list expands all the time.

In the private sector, drug screening gained extensive publicity with the announcement of mandatory testing of professional athletes on baseball and football teams. Other industries implemented drug testing as a screen for job applicants and as a deterrent for drug use among employees. According to the National Institute on Drug Abuse, nearly 30 percent of America's Fortune 500 corporations tested employees during 1986, an increase of 25 percent from the previous year. Hundreds of other companies are reportedly contemplating some type of drug-testing program.

The rapid proliferation of drug screening created a gold-rush atmosphere in the country's testing laboratories. Sales of testing equipment and supplies mushroomed. Executives of one marketing firm report that sales of drug-testing equipment and supplies during 1980 totaled $25 million. By 1985, this figure had grown to $73 million. They report that sales have expanded at a rate of 22 percent a year (Maugh, 1986).

In 1988, American laboratories processed between 15 million to 20 million drug tests. About half of these were for corporations and the rest for prisons, police, and public drug-treatment programs. Of the corporate tests, 85 percent were for pre-employment screening, costing businesses about $200 million annually. Some experts estimate this figure will reach

$500 million annually by 1991 (Kupfer, 1988). This estimate excludes the millions of military drug tests processed by the U.S. Department of Defense each year.

Enterprising drug-testing entrepreneurs enhance sales by marketing directly to parents. By going to a local pharmacy and paying about $25.00 for a urine specimen bottle, parents can ascertain if their children are taking drugs. All a parent has to do is persuade the teenager to cooperate and then send the urine sample to the lab to be checked for traces of marijuana, cocaine, and other drugs. Results come back within two weeks in a plain white envelope. Sales of "hundreds of thousands" of kits are anticipated (Kahtrowitz, 1986).

Local and national politicians have heightened public interest by disagreeing about solutions to the drug problem and by jostling for public attention. Drugs are easier to talk about than most other issues, such as cuts in defense spending. "Soft on Communism is one thing," a political analyst observed, "but soft on drugs is another. Nobody's willing to be accused of that. So everybody's on the bandwagon and it is rolling lickety-split toward the absurd" (Mann, 1986).

Drug-testing hyperbole infused the 1988 election campaigns nationwide. One candidate offered a plan for testing all the nation's high school students and punishing users with mandatory jail sentences. An incumbent governor challenged his opponent to prove he was drug free by submitting to urine tests; both candidates and their wives did so. Even Harold Stassen, the perpetual presidential candidate, now in his ninth decade, reportedly took and passed a urine test. "Next to accepting a campaign contribution from Jane Fonda," one analyst observed, "it seems about the most controversial thing a politician can do these days is refuse his opponent's challenge to take a drug test" (Gailey, 1986). "People seem to think that if you're not for drug testing, you must be for drugs," one observer noted (Newman, 1987).

Political cartoonists and pundits have had a field day with drug-testing in general. "Pissing matches," "jar wars," and "drawing the bottle lines" exemplify their eye-catching captions. They have labeled drug-testing announcements as, "Message from the Bottle," "Testing the Waters," and "Stampede to the Urinals," to cite a few. These pundits refer to the complex guidelines for federal drug testing as a combination of "BIG BROTHER and high school bathroom monitors—a sort of BIG JOHN" (*Time*, March 2, 1987). Critics have labeled drug testers "bladder-cops" and advised employees, "Don't drop your zipper for the gipper" (Gillespie, 1987).

Opponents of drug testing, recommending education, counseling, and other forms of public and employee assistance programs to deal with drug abuse, advance a variety of arguments (O'Keffe, 1987). Urine testing, they say, gives employers a window into the private lives of their employees, revealing hundreds of details about their medical histories, which diseases they are susceptible to, even what they eat and drink. Screening techniques can reveal whether someone has had venereal disease, epilepsy, or mental illness, whether pregnant or predisposed to heart attacks or sickle cell anemia. Because drugs like marijuana can stay for days in the body, drug tests provide employers with information about employees' activities off the job. Meanwhile, these same companies may tolerate or even encourage alcohol consumption as an everyday part of living.

Critics claim that urine testing violates the constitutional protection against unreasonable search and seizure. By monitoring off-the-job behavior it can be a potential instrument of harassment. In America, they say, citizens are presumed to be innocent until proven guilty, not vice versa. Invading the privacy of the many who are innocent to discover the few who are guilty establishes a dangerous and unconstitutional precedent. Observed one critic: "You don't take drugs; you have nothing to hide; but you wouldn't want a tap on your phone. And you don't want a tap on your urine either" (Cohen, 1987).

Drug testing is labeled "an Orwellian nightmare" by one opponent, and "Chemical McCarthyism" by another, "a sinister form of disguised social control." It is "the loyalty oaths of the '80s," one asserted; "drugs are the communism of the decade" (Gillespie, 1987). Referring to drug testing as "a witch hunt," the head toxicologist in North Carolina's Office of the Chief Medical Examiner said, "I am not a communist but I find it hard to criticize communist countries or totalitarian states when I see the kinds of things going on here" (Chapman, 1985).

Voluntary drug testing, critics argue, may be a more ominous evil than mandatory testing. "Giving an individual the right to refuse makes the act of urinating into a bottle a patriotic gesture—a test of your right-mindedness as well as your clean-bloodedness," one observer noted. "The notion of voluntary drug testing is nonsense. If you are using drugs and the test is truly voluntary, you won't take it. The test is meaningless unless the authorities are willing to draw some negative conclusions from a person's refusal to take it. And if they are, it isn't really voluntary, is it?" (*New Republic,* 195, 1986).

Abuses in drug testing have been widely publicized (Weiss, 1986). In 1984, for example, the Georgia Power Company implemented a special hotline for employees to report anonymously the names of drug-abusing colleagues. "Hotlined" employees were then ordered in for a urine test. One employee described her experience like this: Forced to drop her pants, bend over at the waist with her knees slightly bent, she was to hold her right arm in the air, and with her left hand angle a specimen bottle between her legs. Humiliated and embarrassed, she sobbed, shook, wet herself, and vomited. She was fired for insubordination when she refused a second test.

Critics have leveled a plethora of charges against the reliability of urinalysis. "Employers have jumped forward to do urine testing when we don't have the technology to do it accurately," a professor of pharmacology observed (Bloch, 1986). The presence of medicines such as cold remedies and allergy pills, for example, can reportedly cause a person to test positive for marijuana or other drugs. "False positives" can occur because seemingly harmless substances have molecular structures similar to illegal drugs. Painkillers containing ibuprofen can be mistaken for marijuana. Cold, cough, and weight-control medicines containing phenylpropanolamine can be mistaken for amphetamines, and some herbal teas may test like cocaine. A urinalysis may also pick up traces of codeine, commonly used in prescription cough medicines, and amphetamines, which are found in over-the-counter and prescription cold and asthma medications.

Moreover, any chemical test may be unreliable owing to nonstandardized quality-control techniques. For example, an internal military investigation uncovered negligent practices in its own lab testing, leaving in doubt the results of 46,000 positive urine samples taken during 1982 and 1983. Consequently, the U.S. Army reportedly reviewed claims made by any discharged or penalized soldiers who alleged that they were wrongly labeled as drug users during that time. The federal Centers for Disease Control studied thirteen large laboratories that analyzed urine samples for drug-treatment centers. The results showed that, largely because of human error, all of the labs performed unsatisfactorily. They failed to identify correctly even half the samples for four-fifths of the drugs tested. This review, however, concentrated primarily on methadone drug-testing programs and not employee drug testing. The technologies were different as well as the prior probabilities of certain drugs being present.

More recent studies of commercial laboratories (Davis, Hawks, & Blanke, 1988; Frings, Battaglia, & White, 1989) show that urine drug testing can be accurate when the following conditions are met: the tests are performed by a qualified staff who use up-to-date screening and confirmation methods, and there are appropriate quality-control measures and chain of custody. "We do not wish to imply," the researchers state, "that all laboratories accepting employee drug screening specimens are doing inaccurate work. Our study shows, however, that technology and methods are available for accurate drug testing" (Frings, Battaglia, & White, 1989).

Organized approaches to cheating adversely affect reliability problems. A group of San Diego civil libertarians reportedly put together a three-minute telephone tape offering advice on how to disguise drug traces in urine. "Two large tablespoons of bleach poured into a urine sample will help beat the test," a female voice tells callers. "Remember, you have the Constitution on your side" (*Time,* November 20, 1986).

A black market in clean urine has emerged; a vial can sell for as much as $50.00. Selected media show advertisements for such products. One entrepreneur, who formerly sold used cars for a living, reports receiving about a thousand orders during a three-month period. "Sure, it's funny," he said. "We laugh all the way to the bank. It's a pure product, as far as we're concerned; people can wash their cars with it. This is free enterprise." Another entrepreneur, calling himself "The Urine King," sells for $24.95 powdered samples—add water—and a booklet entitled *Success in Urine Testing.* "We are the oldest purveyors of fine urine in the country," he advertises (Collins, 1987).

Critics of drug testing have taken their case to the courts with some success. For example, in 1987, a San Francisco jury awarded damages of $485,000 to a thirty-seven-year-old computer programmer for the Southern Pacific Transportation Company because the company fired her for refusing to take a surprise urinalysis. Her claim relied on a right-to-privacy provision in the California State Constitution. This made companies wary of unannounced random tests and encouraged more careful planning of drug-testing policies.

The testing of job applicants also came under challenge as prospective employees filed suit against companies for invading their privacy (Hafner & Garland, 1988).

A Stanford University athlete (a diver) brought suit against the National Collegiate Athletic Association (NCAA) because the NCAA requires drug testing for intercollegiate competition. The county superior court judge ruled that the association's mandatory drug-testing plan implemented in 1986 for postseason competition was an unconstitutional invasion of privacy. However, the judge allowed limited testing in football and men's basketball because these two sports accounted for all thirty-four athletes who tested positive. Among 3,511 athletes tested, twenty-six tested positive for steroid use, seven for cocaine, and one for amphetamines. "The paradox of this testing program," the judge concluded, "is that a criminal accused of the most serious crimes is afforded more rights than are athletic heroes."

Elaborating on this issue, a sports journalist observed: "Our athletic heroes, once thought to be the stuff that dreams were made of, have lately been reduced to standing before the NCAA's cadre of toilet monitors . . . and urinating into containers. It is the NCAA's conviction that only through this inelegant rite, in which the cup is replenished by the many to atone for the sins of a few, can college athletes once again be purified" (Newman, 1987).

In its first action regarding workplace urinalysis and blood testing, the U.S. Supreme Court ruled by a 7 to 2 vote that it was constitutional for the federal Railroad Administration to test train crews that are involved in accidents. By a less decisive 5 to 4 vote, the High Court ruled in favor of a Customs Service policy of testing applicants for drug-enforcement jobs. Writing for the majority in both cases, Judge Anthony M. Kennedy agreed that blood and urine tests are searches under the Fourth Amendment but cited "special needs" for public safety. The nation has "compelling interests" in keeping drugs out of the country, he asserted. Both experience and common sense suggest that threats of firing employees who use drugs on the job "cannot serve as an effective deterrent unless violators know that they are likely to be discovered."

Dissenting comments by Justice Antonin Scalia in the first case included the warning that "acceptance of dragnet . . . testing ensures that the first and worst casualties of the war on drugs will be the precious liberties of our citizens" (*Newsweek,* April 3, 1989).

The U.S. Attorney General hailed the majority ruling as a momentous victory for the government's drug-testing policy but acknowledged that the administration will have to "tailor its programs to fit the rules" now set by the Supreme Court on who may be tested. At the time of this writing, about forty lawsuits are already pending in federal courts.

In short, there is much about drug testing that is debatable and problematic. The issues are provocative and the implications profound.

This book is neither a scientific monograph nor an encyclopedia of facts and references. Neither is it a technical manual for pharmacologists, laboratory technicians, or forensic experts. Rather, it is written for a more general audience: substance-abuse professionals, educators, and executives of public and private organizations, and secondarily, for parents and employees. In short, it is intended for all those who are affected by drug abuse and who desire to understand the intricacies of the continuing drug-testing saga.

Drug testing is a complex and multifaceted story, and this book approaches the topic from a variety of perspectives: historical, legal, ethical, pharmacological, sociopolitical, sociocultural, and psychosocial.

In Chapter 1, Deborah Ackerman places drug testing in historical perspective. She describes the convergence of a sociocultural problem (drug abuse) with technological advances that have made it possible to detect drugs in urine specimens. The politics of drug testing are discussed in Chapter 2 by J. Michael Walsh and Jeanne G. Trumble. In their review, the authors explore in chronological order the development of arguments, both for and against drug testing; thus, they review the thinking of both advocates and opponents.

In Chapter 3, Ronald M. Paolino summarizes the pharmacology of commonly abused drugs, including information on routes of administration, interactions, and symptoms of use and abuse. Chapter 4, by Robert E. Willette, describes the techniques of drug analysis—that is, chromatography and immunoassay. He offers guidelines on selecting appropriate drug-testing procedures and a competent laboratory.

The next three chapters present the social and cultural contexts of drug testing. In Chapter 5, Paul J. Mulloy recounts the experience of the U.S. Navy in establishing its drug-testing program, which has become a model for such programs in other branches of the government and in private industry. Eric D. Zemper in Chapter 6 discusses drug testing in amateur and professional sports. He makes special reference to the distinction between performance-enhancing drugs and street drugs. In Chapter 7, Helen Axel summarizes results of a national survey of major U.S. corporations, their responses to the problem of employee drug abuse, and efforts to institute drug testing and treatment programs.

In Chapter 8, Robert T. Angarola reviews the legal issues involved in setting up and maintaining drug-testing programs, with reference to recent court decisions. Bernard Lo (Chapter 9) examines the ethical issues regarding drug testing. He discusses when testing is appropriate and looks at standards used to judge such programs. The last two chapters deal with psychosocial issues. Chapter 10, by Robert H. Coombs, addresses the effect of drug testing on mandatory participants. Chapter 11, by Ronald M. Paolino, which concludes this text, explores how employers and others can counsel and help individuals identified through drug testing.

We hope that by telling the story of drug testing, if only the early episodes, this book may enlighten and clarify the national debate. May all who read it find it a valuable resource.

REFERENCES

Applebome, P. (1986, September 30). Plan for school drug testing divides texas town. *The New York Times*, p. A16.

Big John (guidelines for administering drug tests to federal workers). (1987, March 3) *Time*, p. 31.

Bloch, J. (1986, August 11). So what? Everybody's doing it. *Forbes*, p. 102.

Collins, D. (1987, February 23). Drug test fakery: Free enterprise rushes to fill a delicate need. *U.S. News & World Report*, p. 10.

Chapman, F.S. (1985, May). The ruckus over medical testing. *Fortune*, p. 58.

Cohen, N. (1987, May). Editorial. *Sport*, p. 6.

Davis, K.H., Hawks, R.L., & Blanke, R.V. (1988). Assessment of laboratory quality in urine drug testing. *JAMA, 260*, 1749–1754.

Frings, C.S., Battaglia, D.J., & White, R.M. (1989). Status of drugs-of-abuse testing in urine under blind conditions: An AACC study. *Clinical Chemistry, 35*, 891–894.

Gailey, P. (1986, October 12). Drug test challenge. *The New York Times*, p. 31.

Gillespie, E. (1987, December 18). Don't drop your zipper for the gipper. *New Statesman*, p. XIX.

Hafner, K., & Garland, S. (1988, March 28). Testing for drug use: Handle with care. *Business Week*, p. 65.

Kantrowitz, B. (1986, July 21). Bringing home the drug-test dilemma. *Newsweek*, p. 56.

Kelley, J. (1989, December 13). Poll: On-the-job drug use is 'significant'. *USA Today*, p. 1.

Kaufman, I.R. (1986, October 19). The battle over drug testing. *The New York Times*, p. 52.

Kupfer, A. (1988, December 19). Is drug testing good or bad? *Fortune*, pp. 133–134.

Lunzer, F. (1987, July 13). But I've never used drugs. *Forbes*, p. 442.

Mann, J. (1986, September 24). Politician's handy drug war. *Washington Post*, p. C3.

Maugh, T.H. (1986, October 28). Soaring demand erodes drug test lab's efficiency. *Los Angeles Times*, p. 1.

Newman, B. (1987, December 7). Another NCAA fumble. *Sports Illustrated*, p. 100.

O'Keefe, A.M. (1987, June). The case against drug testing. *Psychology Today,* pp. 34–38.

Testing the waters. (1986, November 10). *Time,* p. 35.

The high court weighs drug tests. (1989, April 3). *Newsweek,* p. 8.

TRB from Washington: The right spirit. drugs and family values. (1986, September 8). *New Republic,* p. 4.

Weiss, P. (1986, June). Watch out, urine trouble. *Harper's,* pp. 56–57.

DRUG TESTING

1

A History of Drug Testing

DEBORAH L. ACKERMAN

Drug-testing programs are a fairly recent attempt to solve the problem of widespread substance abuse and its consequences. In the early 1960s urine testing for drugs was a technique used exclusively in methadone maintenance, in drug rehabilitation programs, and in other clinical settings. But mandatory testing for other substances of abuse reached another segment of the U.S. population in the late 1960s when the International Olympic Committee banned a number of substances used by athletes to improve performance. About the same time, the U.S. Department of Defense introduced mandatory urine screening to detect heroin use among military personnel returning from Vietnam. And by the late 1970s, law enforcement agencies had begun to employ urine testing in the jails to control and monitor the criminal activity of drug-dependent individuals. It was not until the early 1980s that the first mass screening program was introduced by the military services. This program was facilitated by the development and refinement of low-cost, efficient techniques to detect a large number of drugs in a single urine specimen and was motivated by concern in the military that widespread drug use would interfere with operational readiness and safety. A similar concern among U.S. government and private employers has led, most recently, to the extension of mandatory drug testing into the workplace.

Throughout history, in every society, people have used drugs, not only to cure illness and alleviate pain, but also to alter mood, thought, and feeling and to improve physical and mental performance. Furthermore, there have always been individuals and groups whose use of drugs has deviated from the medical and social conventions of the time. Societies express their disapproval of such aberrant behavior by calling it "drug abuse." Because the definition of drug abuse is culturally determined, the behaviors and drugs so labeled vary considerably from culture to culture and within the same culture from time to time. In contemporary society, such deviant behavior may range from self-experimentation or the occasional use of alcohol or marijuana to compulsive drug taking, in which individuals behave as though they cannot function optimally without certain drugs. Self-experimentation, arising from natural curiosity or a need to conform to one's peer group, is better tolerated. On the other hand, compulsive drug use is seen as harmful to both the individual and to society, and legal constraints have been established to protect both.

Mandatory drug testing is contemporary society's response to what is currently defined as drug abuse. It is a relatively recent event that represents the convergence of two separate phenomena: the current epidemic of drug abuse and the evolution of the technology that makes it possible to detect drugs in biological specimens. To tell the history of drug testing requires, therefore, a review of both its sociocultural and technological antecedents.[1]

PRIOR TO 1900

Drug Abuse and Attempts to Control It

The first substance acknowledged for its ability to foster dependence, and thus for its abuse potential, was alcohol. References to the "drinking habit" can be found in the Bible and in the writings of ancient physicians. Plato advised that wine be prohibited to children, slaves, and magistrates (*Laws* 2:674 a,b), and the New Testament warns that those who engage in drunkenness shall not inherit the Kingdom of God (Galatians 5:21).

The earliest legal constraints on alcohol date back to ancient Babylon. The Code of Hammurabi restricted wine sales, forbade priestesses from entering wine shops, and controlled prices. There are tales that in China royal astronomers were put to death for being drunk and missing an eclipse. In Persia, heavy drinkers were led through the streets by a cord strung through their noses; persistent offenders were tied with a nose cord to a stake in the public square. During the Middle Ages in China and Japan, various temperance decrees were promulgated by a succession of emperors who limited the manufacture, sale, and consumption of wine and saki. Despite such measures, alcohol use and abuse flourished in most cultures and throughout all social strata.

Between the sixteenth and eighteenth centuries, following the introduction of the more potent and more disruptive distilled spirits, controls on excessive alcohol consumption were based on both religious and economic principles; however, economic controls met with public and private opposition. In Europe, religious reformers were concerned about the morality of alcohol abuse and called for moderation or total abstinence. Later, Puritan reformers in the United States inveighed against alcoholic vice. In England, Edward VI first attempted to control the acquisition of alcohol by enacting a law requiring licensure of alehouses. Subsequent measures to control retail sales of alcohol by excise taxes, licenses, and prohibitions resulted in bootlegging and violence (i.e., the "Gin Riots") and forced their repeal. While in the United States, the Whiskey Rebellion of 1794, in which revenue officers who tried to enforce the excise law of 1791 were tarred and feathered by angry locals, demonstrated to the government the unpopularity of attempts to regulate sales of alcoholic beverages.

In the nineteenth century, concern for the adverse effects of alcohol on the individual, combined with concern for society, fueled several attempts at prohibition. Physicians such as Benjamin Rush had begun to consider the medical consequences of alcohol abuse. And, of course, the temperance movement gained supporters and influence throughout the century. In 1827 the American Society for the Promotion of Temperance was founded. In 1851 the first prohibition law was enacted in Maine, and within four years, thirteen states had similar statutes. However, by 1870, most states had either repealed the laws or significantly modified them. At the end of the nineteenth century a second wave of prohibition and the efforts of Carry Nation resulted in new laws, the majority of which were again repealed within a few years.

During the same period, other substances began to be regarded as harmful to both the individual and to society. Such drugs as opium, which had been a problem in China for many years, and morphine, cocaine, and heroin were recognized as addictive. Opium had been used in western Asia and the Mediterranean as an analgesic and hypnotic for as long as alcohol had been used. The practice of eating opium spread to other parts of the world, and a lucrative trade in opium exporting was well established by the nineteenth century. In China, where opium smoking became the preferred mode of ingestion, attempts were made to control the addiction. By the early 1800s the Chinese government had tried numerous prohibitions, taxation, and the banning of imports, yet the ranks of opium addicts increased. Some addicts migrated to the West, bringing opium with them. Americans curious for new experiences began to experiment with opium, and opiates as unregulated additives in syrups and elixirs were readily available to the public. Dependency and withdrawal symptoms alarmed both health officials and the general public.

When morphine was isolated in the early 1800s it was heralded for its potent analgesic properties. However, after the Civil War a population of morphine-addicted veterans emerged, and morphine became a drug to be feared. By the end of the century, when heroin was introduced, it was used to relieve opium withdrawal symptoms, but soon heroin addiction replaced opium addiction. Cocaine, first lauded as both a local anesthetic and as a cure for morphine addiction, aroused alarm as the numbers of addicts—including physicians, artists, and others—grew. Gradually the United States began to realize it had a drug problem, and before the end of the century, several states adopted laws prohibiting opium smoking, and measures to control the other drugs were considered.

Although cannabis had been used for centuries in Asia for religious ceremonies, it was not considered a threat to Western nations until the late eighteenth century. Cannabis, in the form of hashish, had first gained a bad reputation in the late eleventh century because of its association with the assassins of what is now Iran and Iraq. At that time, Hasan-i-Sabba, the Old Man of the Mountain, used hashish to motivate his band of murderous raiders, who became known as "assassins" for "hashih eaters." Following the introduction of tobacco and the technique of smoking dried leaves, marijuana use began to spread slowly throughout the Eastern Hemisphere and across the ocean.

Drug Detection

As society formulated its notion of drug abuse, as it expanded the list of drugs of abuse, and as it introduced laws to control the use of those drugs, there were no techniques in place to identify individual drug users. Their actions to buy or sell drugs, or while under a drug's influence, and such physiological signs as constricted pupils caused by narcotic intoxication were all that authorities could rely on to identify users.

Although physicians had long recognized the utility of urinalysis as an aid to diagnosis, the technology had not yet been developed to detect drugs in urine. Haber (1988) has suggested that urinalysis may be the oldest of all laboratory tests. Haber cites Hippocrates, who believed that urine was a filtrate of the blood, as the first to recommend examining the urine to help make a medical diagnosis. The practice of visually examining the urine was continued and elaborated upon until the late 1500s, when it fell out of favor. Eventually, by the nineteenth century, after technological advances made chemical and microscopic analyses possible, urinalysis came to be a standard diagnostic aid. And while it was also known that most drugs leave the body either unchanged or as metabolites in urine, the specific techniques for detecting them were still unavailable.

FROM THE TURN OF THE CENTURY
TO THE 1950s

Drug Abuse and Attempts to Control It

After the turn of the century, the U.S. government began to heed the growing public concern about drug and alcohol abuse. Congress passed the Pure Food and Drug Act of 1906, which required that warning labels be added to prescription medications containing substances known to be habit-forming. The importation of smokable opium was banned in 1909, and restrictions on prescription drugs tightened with the passage of the Harrison Act in 1914. This act severely limited the sale of narcotics and required physicians and pharmacists to maintain records of drugs dispensed and prescribed, so that the government could monitor the distribution of narcotics. Additional laws prohibited the importation of these drugs, which resulted in the creation of a narcotics underground.

By 1919 the temperance movement had gained enough popular support to force passage of the 18th Amendment to the U.S. Constitution. Rather than curtail excessive drinking, however, the era of Prohibition merely effected a change in drinking behavior from socially and legally accepted patterns to illegal and covert use. But by 1933, after fourteen years, the experiment with Prohibition ended. Ironically in the following year, Alcoholics Anonymous was formed.

Marijuana use spread in the first half of this century. Tincture of cannabis was available by prescription as an analgesic and hypnotic. Although marijuana was not widely smoked except by certain ethnic groups and others who, during Prohibition, found it easier to obtain than alcohol, it became the subject of journalistic sensationalism. Marijuana was described as the first step to heroin and as leading to insanity and murder. Such reports aroused the public and resulted in the enactment in 1937 of the Marihuana Tax Act. This legislation levied a token tax with harsh penalties for failure to pay on all who prescribed or possessed it, and established marijuana as a dangerous drug.

The first half of the twentieth century brought many developments in medicinal chemistry—and many new substances with abuse potential. Naturally occurring stimulants and hallucinogens were isolated and purified, and other psychoactive drugs were synthesized. Barbital was introduced in 1903, spawning the synthesis of many other barbiturates, and in the 1920s various naturally occurring and synthetic stimulants were introduced. About the same time, scientists became interested in the psychoactive properties of peyote cactus and mushrooms that had been used for centuries by natives of the Southwestern United States and Mexico. Following Albert Hoffman's discovery in 1943 of the psychedelic effects of LSD, clinical interest was sparked by the belief that such drug effects might be related to the biochemistry of mental illness, and thus help to create effective therapeutics.

Drug Detection

With advances in drug isolation, purification, and synthesis came the development of techniques to detect and quantify drugs in urine and other biologic specimens. The oldest technique for detecting drugs or their metabolites in urine is solvent extraction. Solvent extraction was employed to extract selectively acidic and basic drugs by adjusting the acidity of the solvent. Various chromatographic methods were developed to separate compounds and identify components based on their unique abilities to interact with fixed (immobile) substances (adsorption). Lederer (1989) cited Goppelsroeder's 1904 book *Studien uber die Anwendung der Capillaranalyse* as marking the introduction of chromatography in the medical sciences. Subsequent refinements in the choice of solvents and adsorbents made the techniques more powerful. Paper chromatography, available in 1944, enabled the successful diagnostic differentiation of a number of metabolic diseases through urinalysis. Additional methods that depend upon substances' unique abilities to absorb and emit light were developed and used to detect specific drugs such as heroin, morphine, and cocaine.

The first drug-screening program was introduced in the early 1920s, but it was not based on urinalysis. It was established to detect alcohol intoxication. Because alcohol is quickly metabolized and excreted primarily through the lungs, determination of alcohol ingestion must be made by analyzing blood or breath. During Prohibition, blood samples from motorists charged with driving while intoxicated were submitted for crude biochemical analysis. Within ten years the noninvasive breath analyzers replaced blood-testing kits (Montagne, Pugh, & Fink, 1988).

FROM 1950 TO THE PRESENT

Drug Abuse and Attempts to Control It

In the second half of the twentieth century, legislation broadened to include new classes of drugs that earlier were not believed to have much abuse potential. For example, hallucinogenic chemicals were not considered drugs of abuse when scientists studied their psychological, biological, and behavioral effects, or when small groups of college students experimented with them. However, as experimentation became more widespread, their use became "abuse." Thus, by the end of the 1960s, legal constraints were introduced for their possession, manufacture, or sale. Also newer drugs such as phencyclidine (PCP) gained popularity. PCP had been developed in the 1950s as a surgical anesthetic because of its dissociative effects, but it was abandoned, except in veterinary medicine, because of adverse effects such as delirium and hallucinations. These same effects, and the fact that it can be synthesized in underground laboratories, made it attractive to illicit drug users. PCP soon reappeared on the streets. Most recently, so-called designer drugs have appeared. They resemble narcotics but may be many times more potent, more toxic, and more addictive. Because they are manufactured in underground laboratories, they are more difficult to control.

In the 1960s an "epidemic" of drug abuse began as American middle and upper class youth started experimenting with marijuana, LSD, and other hallucinogens. This same group increasingly began to use drugs known to cause dependency, including cocaine, heroin, and stimulants. Winick (1973) attributes the increase in drug abuse that occurred in the 1960s to a number of social and economic influences. Among them were the Vietnam War, the high proportion of young people in the population ("baby boomers"), the media's highlighting of substance use, and the efforts by government to implement a war on crime with an anti-drug crusade. A survey by the National Commission on Marihuana and Drug Abuse (1973) found that substantial percentages of American youth and adults had reported experience with marijuana (14 and 16 percent, respectively), LSD and other hallucinogens (4.8 and 4.6 percent), and (nonmedical use of) sedatives, tranquilizers, and stimulants (15 and 22 percent). More youth than adults had sniffed glue and other inhalants (6.4 compared with 2.1 percent), while more adults had experience with cocaine (3.2 compared with 1.5 percent) and heroin (1.3 compared with 0.6 percent).

The growing use of illicit drugs, especially among the young, prompted the strongest legislation to date—the Controlled Substances Act, which Congress passed in 1971. This legislation superseded both the Harrison Act and the 1956 Narcotic Control Act. It divided drugs into five categories based on addictive properties and medical usefulness, and it required pharmacists to keep records for two years of all controlled substances dispensed. Additional requirements spelled out the manner in which prescriptions are prepared and renewed. While such legislation is effective in controlling the dispensing of many substances, it cannot control the many drugs that are synthesized in underground laboratories and sold on the street (Swinyard, 1985).

A number of surveys on drug abuse revealed that over the next decade the overall use of illicit substances had increased but that consumption patterns had changed. Data compiled through the National Household Survey on Drug Abuse (NIDA, 1982) showed that marijuana use had peaked in 1979 and remained higher in 1982 than in 1972 for youth but not for young adults; hallucinogen use was lower for both groups in 1982 after having peaked in 1979; heroin use was lower for both groups, having peaked in 1975; but the use of cocaine, other stimulants, and sedatives increased throughout the interval for both groups.

A study was conducted in 1980 by NIDA to project drug abuse among young adults in future years (Richards, 1981). Projections were based on demographic trends and survey data on the nonmedical use of drugs. The final report used consumption rates for the year 1977 and assumed that they would remain the same through 1995. It concluded that regular use of marijuana would increase but occasional use would stabilize; hallucinogen, heroin, and other opiate use would not change dramatically; and that cocaine use would increase. The report added that these projections should be interpreted cautiously because they do not account for other significant sociological and demographic trends, and the assumption that current trends would continue may be misleading.

West and Cohen (1985) have suggested that current drug use may be more harmful than in the past. The drugs of the second half of the twentieth century are more potent and better purified than the naturally occurring substances of the nineteenth and early twentieth centuries. The introduction of numerous synthetic drugs, as well as the tendency of many people to abuse multiple drugs, has added to the danger. Additional causes of concern are the earlier age of onset of drug use, the increase in the proportion of females using drugs, including pregnant women, and the multiple lines of supplies. Concerns that current drug abuse is more widespread and that the drugs themselves (and the dependency they foster) are substantially more harmful to individuals and to society as a whole have sparked more intensive preventive efforts and interventions.

In March 1986, the President's Commission on Organized Crime recommended that all employees of private companies contracting with the federal government be regularly subjected to urine testing for drugs as a condition of employment. In September 1986, President Ronald Reagan issued an Executive Order that called for the establishment of a drug-free federal workplace and for the mass drug testing of federal employees in "sensitive" positions. The next year Congress passed the Supplemental Appropriations Act of 1987 as an attempt to establish uniform drug-testing programs among the various federal agencies.

Drug Detection

The techniques that make it possible to conduct mass screening programs have been developed only since the 1950s. (See, for example, reviews by Kaistha, 1972; Decker, 1977; Hawks, 1986; and Willette, this volume.) Numerous chromatographic methods and their applications evolved during this period. Paper chromatography, which had been introduced in the 1940s, was used in the early 1960s to screen for amphetamines in urine, and by the late 1960s it was used to detect barbiturates. Also in the 1960s column absorption chromatography methods were developed to separate and purify narcotics, heroin, and barbiturates. By the late 1960s thin-layer chromatography (TLC) had become the most widely used technique. It is inexpensive, relatively rapid, and permits the simultaneous detection of a wide range of substances in a single test run. Its sensitivity can be easily adapted for the purpose of the screening. Gas chromatography (GC) appeared in the late 1960s to identify and quantify narcotics, cocaine, codeine, barbiturates, and stimulants. Almost all drugs are amenable to GC analysis. When coupled with mass spectrometry (GC-MS) in the 1970s it could detect and identify all drugs of abuse in biologic specimens.

The most recent methodologies developed in the 1970s are the immunoassays: free radical immunoassay (FRAT), hemagglutination inhibition (HI), enzyme-multiplied inhibition assay (EMIT), and radioimmunoassay (RIA). EMIT assays currently are being marketed as tests to be performed on-site by personnel not primarily trained as laboratory workers. They are available in a variety of kits for screening urine for amphetamines, barbiturates, benzodiazepines, cocaine metabolites, methadone, phencyclidine, morphine, propoxyphene, ethanol, and urinary metabolites of marijuana.

In clinical settings urine testing for drug use has been a routine procedure especially in emergencies when drug intake is suspected. In the mid-1970s screening was recommended as an aid to proper diagnosis of psychiatric outpatients. It was seen as the simplest and most efficient tool for the diagnosis of substance abuse. Screening procedures were recommended to evaluate new patients on admission and when there was diagnostic confusion (Hall et al., 1977, 1978). As drug abuse increased and more and more outpatient and inpatient treatment programs for drug-dependent individuals were established throughout the country, drug screening came to be used routinely to monitor surreptitious drug use.

The military first instituted urine testing to identify heroin users returning from Vietnam in the late 1960s and early 1970s. Because the screening method, FRAT, was being used to detect only morphine (the major metabolite of heroin excreted in urine), other drugs remained undetected. Many returnees, who knew the approximate date when they would return home, were able to pass the test by temporarily switching to methadone, barbiturates, or tranquilizers to get through heroin withdrawal. By the early 1970s the Army had extended its screening program to detect other drugs among soldiers reporting for active duty. Today the military employs mass screening of all enlisted personnel as well as civilian employees in sensitive positions.

Also in the early 1970s a number of pilot programs were introduced to monitor patterns of drug use and the criminal activity of known drug-dependent individuals. The Special Action Office for Drug Abuse Prevention (SAODAP), the Law Enforcement Assistance Administration (LEAA), and the National Institute on Drug Abuse (NIDA) began to sponsor drug-screening programs throughout the country to control the criminal activity of drug-dependent individuals (Cordova & Banford, 1975). One pilot program was sponsored by NIDA to monitor patterns of drug use in given geographic areas by introducing a urine-screening program in the jails (Richardson & Moerin, 1979). Implementation of these programs was made possible by the recent development of analytical methods to detect a variety of drugs in large numbers of specimens.

The choice of a method depends on the need for speed, sensitivity, and specificity, as well as the need to detect a wide variety of drugs and to process a large number of specimens at a reasonable cost. The most sensitive techniques are also the most expensive to employ in detecting a large number of drugs. Currently there are more than 50,000 chemicals, including drugs, used in industry and medicine. If only a small percentage of these had the potential for abuse, the cost of a comprehensive screening program to identify and quantitate them would be prohibitive. Therefore, a drug-screening program also must focus on the drugs and chemicals that are known to be abused within the community being screened.

SPECIFIC DRUG-TESTING PROGRAMS

The Military

The largest mass screening program today is run by the U.S. Navy (see Mulloy, this volume). The Navy's program was initiated after a 1980 Pentagon survey, conducted through anonymous questionnaires among 20,000 military personnel, showed that 27 percent of Navy personnel under the age of twenty-five were using drugs. Another impetus was the May 1981 crash of a Marine Corps aircraft aboard the aircraft carrier *Nimitz*. Six of the ten deck crew members who died had used illegal drugs within the previous thirty days.

When the Navy's program was instituted, the four laboratories that were to perform the urine tests were overwhelmed with samples before the labs were adequately staffed to handle them. Some laboratories took shortcuts, such as confirming a positive result by using the same testing procedure as the initial detection method. More serious problems were the result of accidental contamination and improper identification. By the end of the first year of testing, breaches in proper handling of specimens cast doubt on positive samples taken from some 4,500 individuals. Disciplinary action against 1,034 Navy personnel had to be reversed (Maugh, 1986).

These events led to the appointment of a special commission under the leadership of Major General David Einsel to investigate the problems. The Einsel Commission Report, released in 1984, told of a devastating error rate that was attributed not to the tests themselves but to poor management, inadequate personnel, broken chain of custody, and faulty record keeping. The report has been criticized by Morgan (1984) for its failure to find false positives in view of statements made by the former commander of one of the laboratories that estimated a false-positive rate of 3 to 5 percent because of contaminated glassware. Morgan also took issue with the report because it recommended that confirmation of false positives be made through gas chromatography alone, which may be inaccurate, rather than through GC-MS.

Today the Navy's program is considered a paradigm with rigorous laboratory procedures and built-in safeguards to ensure reliable results. In 1985 only eleven disciplinary actions were reversed because of laboratory errors or improper handling of specimens (Maugh, 1986). The Navy has five labs that perform some 1.8 million urinalysis a year, or about three specimens for each Navy member. The labs use radioimmunoassays to screen for amphetamines, barbiturates, cocaine, marijuana, opiates, and PCP. All positive test results are then confirmed by gas chromatography/ mass spectrometry. In addition, proficiency testing of laboratories is performed weekly. Drug programs in the other branches of the military are operated in much the same manner, but they are less extensive.

Amateur Athletics

In sports and athletics the rationale behind mandatory drug testing has evolved over time. Drug testing began as an intervention to remove any unfair advantage that an athlete who uses drugs might have. This reason was especially valid for drugs such as central nervous system (CNS) stimulants and (later) anabolic steroids—two groups of drugs that are believed to improve physical performance and endurance. The banning of analgesics, which can mask the pain of an injury and can lead to more serious injury, was motivated by a desire to protect athletes from the potentially dangerous drug side effects. Today, drug testing serves additionally as a primary intervention to discourage children and adolescents from using street drugs. In this context, "clean" athletes serve as role models to prevent the youth of today from becoming tomorrow's addicts, and to promote a drug-free society.

Although drugs have been used by athletes to enhance performance ever since the first Olympic Games were played (the Greeks of antiquity are believed to have used psychoactive mushrooms to improve *their* performance), the first mandatory drug-testing programs were not introduced until 1968 by the International Olympic Committee (IOC). Even in the modern games, various stimulants have been used. During the 1904 Olympics in St. Louis, marathon winner Thomas Hicks was believed to have been aided by a cocktail of strychnine, a stimulant, and brandy. Similar reports about competitors' surreptitious drug use continued. At the 1960 Summer Olympic Games in Rome, Danish cyclist Kurt Jensen was killed after taking amphetamines and a vasodilator. In response, a series of conferences were held to address the problem of "doping" in sports. (The term "doping" has been attributed to the Kaffirs of southeastern Africa who used a liquor called *dop* as a stimulant.) The result of these conferences was the implementation of spot checks at the 1964 Olympic Games in Tokyo and the introduction of formal testing for stimulants at the 1968 Winter and Summer Olympic Games (Puffer, 1986). Three years later, a report by the Medical Commission of the British Commonwealth Games Federation, which had instituted similar regulations, concluded that the introduction of random testing had greatly reduced the use of stimulants (Prevention and Detection of Drug Taking ['doping'] at the IX British Commonwealth Games, 1971).

The first major controversy over drug testing occurred in 1972 during the Summer Olympics in Munich. American swimmer Rick DeMont, who suffered from asthma, was stripped of his gold medal because traces of the stimulant ephedrine, an asthma medication, were found in his urine. Following the furor over that case, the IOC subsequently permitted salbutamol, terbutaline, and other bronchodilators at the Montreal Summer Games in 1976.

The IOC introduced testing for anabolic steroids in Montreal. Anabolic steroids are used by some athletes in sports that require strength because they promote the growth of skeletal muscle. In addition to their potential for providing users with a possible unfair advantage, steroids trigger a number of potentially serious adverse effects such as hepatic carcinoma, impotence, and jaundice. While long recognized as drugs of abuse in athletic competition, steroid detection was not possible until the development of reliable analytic technology in the 1970s (Hatton & Catlin, 1987). Of the 275 samples tested in Montreal, 8 were positive. In comparison, only three of 1,786 samples tested positive for the other banned substances (Barnes, 1980). In the preliminaries to the 1980 Moscow Olympics, the top three women's 1,500-meter runners were banned from competition for life by the International Amateur Athletic Federation. All had been found guilty of taking anabolic steroids. At the 1983 Pan American Games in Caracas, thirty athletes, including fifteen medalists, tested positive for drugs, mostly anabolic steroids (Harvey, 1987). Most recently, Canadian sprinter Ben Johnson was stripped of the gold medal earned in the 1988 Summer Olympic Games after testing positive for anabolic steroids.

Currently the IOC bans substances in five categories: psychomotor stimulants, sympathomimetic amines, miscellaneous CNS stimulants, narcotic analgesics, and anabolic steroids. In addition, blood doping and the use of growth hormone (both discussed below) are prohibited.

In January 1986 the National Collegiate Athletic Association (NCAA) initiated its drug-testing program so that, according to its policy statement, no one participant might be pressured to use chemical substances in order to remain competitive. The banned drug list of the NCAA is similar to that of the IOC but also includes a number of substances banned for specific sports, diuretics, and recreational drugs (i.e., cannabis), and does not ban narcotic analgesics. The rules drawn up by the NCAA require that all student athletes sign an annual consent form prior to participating in any sport. The use of several drugs prescribed for the treatment of asthma must be declared before competition, and corticosteroid use must be declared at NCAA championships or certified football games.

The most recent practice of "blood doping," or "blood boosting," has been the subject of debate. Autologous blood boosting entails withdrawing 2 pints of blood from an individual, freezing the red blood cells, and then once the body has replaced the lost blood, returning the thawed cells just before competition. The "boosted" number of red blood cells increases the competitors' oxygen supply. Several studies have indicated that boosting can improve the performance of trained athletes, although the improvement appears to be a slight one. In 1984 in Los Angeles, American cyclist Pat McDonough admitted he had his blood boosted prior to competing. However, McDonough and possibly many other teammates used donor blood (homologous boosting) because the technique was used after it was too late to extract their own blood and still recover in time to compete. Homologous transfusions place healthy subjects at unnecessary risk. Even autologous transfusion may be hazardous if not carried out under careful medical supervision (see the "American College of Sports Medicine position on blood doping as an ergogenic aid," 1987).

Although the practice of blood doping has been banned by both the IOC and the NCAA, to date no analytical method has been devised for unequivocal detection. One method was described recently (Berglund, Hemmingssohn, & Birgegard, 1987), but it can only detect 50 percent of the blood-doped athletes by a single test sample, and according to IOC rules, athletes are required only to submit urine samples.

Growth hormone is a powerful anabolic substance that affects all body systems and plays an important role in muscle growth. It is released from the anterior pituitary gland in response to a variety of stimuli including exercise, sleep, stress, and the administration of a variety of drugs and amino acids. Growth hormone administration to normal animals leads to muscle hypertrophy, but this muscular growth is not accompanied by increased strength. Growth hormone excess leads to acromegaly, a disease with significant morbidity, including a myopathy in which muscles appear larger but are functionally weaker (Murad & Haynes, 1985).

Although there is no scientific evidence that athletic performance is improved by growth hormone supplementation, this practice is becoming more widespread among athletes because it cannot be detected at present. There have been anecdotal reports that some athletes are injecting themselves with cadaveric or biosynthetic forms of growth hormone, both of which are associated with potentially serious complications, and ingesting amino acids in the belief that their endogenous growth hormone secretion will be increased. There have been no studies on the effects of growth hormone supplementation, and the anecdotal reports have been equivocal, with some individuals reporting spectacular results and others reporting no effect. Despite the lack of valid evidence for its efficacy and its potentially serious side effects, growth hormone use may increase. Both its use and abuse have the potential to change dramatically the future conduct of athletics and threaten the concept of fair and honest competition.

The Workplace

Drug and alcohol abuse has been a major challenge confronting American industry. In the 1960s heroin addiction was seen as the greatest threat to the health and safety of American workers. By the early 1970s other drugs of abuse began to be considered threats to industry. These included other opiates, amphetamines, stimulants, and other psychoactive drugs such as marijuana. In 1986 the National Institute on Drug Abuse estimated that the cost to American business of employee drug and alcohol abuse was $100 billion annually (Hawkes & Chiang, 1986).

In the early 1970s Sohn and others (1970, 1972) advocated drug-screening programs to prevent the problems of increased illness and injury caused by addicted employees. Such programs were to be used to detect drug users in pre-employment processing and when there was obvious impairment of work performance. However, mandatory drug testing was to be used only to a limited extent on some individuals who had been involved in on-the-job accidents.

A decade later Cohen (1984) considered compulsory drug screening as a means to reduce the cost of drug abuse to American industry. He cited an estimate by the Metropolitan Life Insurance Company that on-the-job drug use costs industry approximately $85 billion annually in lost time, impaired productivity, and injuries. The three drugs constituting the bulk of the problem were alcohol, marijuana, and cocaine, with heroin and other opiates also being used. Cohen advocated pre-employment screening and offered employers several options to deal with drug use on the job: ignore the problem; adopt a strict disciplinary approach of dismissing employees in highly sensitive positions who use drugs either on the job or before coming to work; or rehabilitate drug users and search out other users among suspected individuals.

Pre-employment drug screening was introduced several years ago in some large corporations and in federal agencies. According to a 1984 survey, 18 percent of Fortune 500 companies conducted some form of urine testing on their employees.[2] The National Institute on Drug Abuse estimates that figure has risen to 40 percent today. A 1988 Gallup survey revealed that 28 percent of the nation's largest companies use drug tests to screen applicants. In 1984, the U.S. Secret Service began an employee drug-screening program to test applicants and probationary officers. By early 1986, several other federal agencies had either initiated or established guidelines for their own screening programs.

A survey of technical experts, arbitrators, and testing laboratories was conducted to evaluate the legal basis of employee drug testing (Hoyt et al., 1987). Investigators found at that time that no consistent methodology or set of criteria for employee drug testing had been established, except in the U.S. military. Both NIDA and the Department of Health and Human Services have only recently drafted guidelines for accreditation of drug-testing laboratories and drug-testing programs ("Mandatory Guidelines for Federal Workplace Drug Testing Programs: Final Guidelines," April 1988). While the Mandatory Guidelines apply to the testing of government employees, they should provide a model for testing in the workplace.

Mandatory drug testing of federal employees was recently upheld by the U.S. Supreme Court. Two cases challenging the government's right to conduct urine testing were decided in March 1989. The decision in the first case (*National Treasury Employees' Union* vs. *von Raab*, 86-1879) upheld the government's right to require urine tests for U.S. Customs Service employees seeking drug-enforcement jobs. In the second case (*Skinner* vs. *Railway Labor Executives' Association*, 87-1555) the Supreme Court upheld mandatory blood and urine tests for railroad workers involved in accidents. In the past, the Court had generally required that there be some evidence implicating an individual before allowing authorities to search for drugs or alcohol. The High Court said that its recent decisions did not violate privacy rights even though there is no such advance evidence.

Two other recent decisions deal with the issue of random drug testing. In both cases (*Guiney* vs. *Roache*, 89-205, and *Policeman's Benevolent Association* vs. *Washington Township*, 88-706) the High Court let stand lower court rulings permitting the random testing of police officers even when there is no reason to suspect drug abuse. These rulings indicate that the justices are willing to allow widespread testing of employees in jobs that affect public safety.

THE CONTROVERSY

In 1972, Lundberg described drug screening as "chemical McCarthyism." Testing, which had previously affected only military personnel, athletes, probation parolees, methadone-program participants, and hospital overdose patients, had begun to be imposed upon business employees and applicants. At that time the existing technology was so imperfect that the performance of even the best toxicology laboratories was grossly defective, with error rates on unknown samples commonly as high as 20 to 70 percent. Yet the results of such screenings were responsible for an employee getting and keeping his job, an addict's freedom, and a soldier's future employability.

Fourteen years later in reexamining the issue of drug screening, Lundberg (1986) wrote that, although urine drug-screening technology had improved immensely, under no circumstances could impairment be diagnosed or even presumed from a urine test result. Lundberg argued that the principal purpose of urine drug screening is legal, not medical. If society feels that the problems of drug abuse are so great as to justify the loss of individual freedom through mandatory random urine tests, then the decision should be made by the electorate, probably through state-by-state referenda.

Morgan (1984) has argued that cost estimates of drug abuse are based on the questionable assumptions that dysfunctional work (or life) and a history of use or the presence of a drug are causally related, and that people who use drugs will inevitably malfunction in a fashion similar to the drug abusers seen in treatment programs. Morgan questioned these assumptions because there is no proven correlation between a positive urine test for drugs and observed or assessed human behavior. The real justification for the screening of urine in industry or elsewhere, Morgan argued, is the identification of deviant, rather than dysfunctional, behavior. Morgan likened drug testing to polygraph tests, which are used to uncover intimate details about the moral behavior of individuals.

The American Medical Association (AMA) has called for the development of tests to detect impairment caused by drug and alcohol use rather than to detect drug use. In 1984 the AMA supported a rule proposed by the Federal Railroad Administration for the control of alcohol and drug abuse in railroad operations. The rule called for toxicologic testing before employment, after accidents, and for reasonable cause, and the establishment of employee assistance programs to treat employees who have a drug or alcohol problem. The following year the AMA recommended to the Federal Aviation Administration (FAA) that a more effective approach would be to develop a method of detecting mental and physical impairments that may result from alcohol and drug abuse or dependence rather than a chemical method of detecting alcohol or drug use. In the same year the AMA's House of Delegates issued a report that opposed employment discrimination based on any health condition not related to the requirements of the job, and suggested that the AMA develop model federal and state legislation that would prohibit such discrimination. Later, the House of Delegates adopted a report by the Council on Scientific Affairs that concluded that drug testing does not provide any information about mental or physical impairments that may be due to drug use or about patterns of abuse (Council on Scientific Affairs, 1987).

It is clear that drug abuse is viewed as such to the extent that it elicits behavior harmful to both the individual and to society. Prior to drug screening, the only way society had to detect an individual's drug dependency was by his or her behavior to procure, possess or profit by drugs, or by the person's behavior while under a drug's influence. Legal constraints on behavior (to possess) were the best society once had to control drug abuse.

Drug screening is a considerable improvement; however, its limitation is that it does not permit the distinction between drug user and drug abuser—occasional, benign use versus compulsive, harmful abuse. At present, that goal is best approached by setting the minimum detectable level at some intermediate level. However, the selection of cut-off level is currently arbitrary. Each individual screening program may set a different level. The military's program, for example, has set the minimum detectable level of marijuana at 100 nanograms (ng) cannabinol per milliliter (mL). A number of state and private employers, such as the Department of Water and Power, Pacific Gas and Electric, and Lockheed Corporation in California, and the Greyhound Company, have done the same. On the other hand, other employers, such as the *Los Angeles Times,* use a level of 50 ng/mL (*Los Angeles Times,* 1986).

Often the damage to society is evaluated in dollars and cents. The rationale for drug-testing programs is expressed in terms of money saved through the prevention of accident-related loss of life and property and by reduced productivity. However, today's screening programs have not been set up to detect the costliest drug of abuse—alcohol. In 1986 NIDA estimated that the annual cost to industry of alcohol use is approximately $67 billion, or twice the cost of nonalcohol drug abuse (Hawks & Chiang, 1986).

Mandatory drug testing is an intervention motivated by two concerns: to protect people from doing harm to themselves and to protect all of us from each other. The former represents a medical problem; the latter, a legal one. Because of this fundamental difference, the solutions to each may not rest in a single best approach. Further, with employees in both the private and public sectors, including athletes, challenging mandatory drug testing, the issue of protecting the rights of the individual (i.e., from government, employers, etc.) has been added. Drug testing has now entered the tug-of-war between private rights and the public good that has been ongoing in this country ever since its founding. Thus, while the history of drug testing in the laboratories has been brief, the history of the legal principles attending it is long. And drug testing's future, at least its immediate future, will be in the courts.

REFERENCES

American College of Sports Medicine position on blood doping as an ergogenic aid. (1987). *Medical Science and Sports Exercise, 19,* 540–543.

Barnes, L. (1980). Olympic drug testing: Improvements without progress. *Physician Sports Medicine, 8*(6), 21–24.

Berglund, B., Hemmingsson, P., & Birgegard, G. (1987). Detection of autologous blood transfusions in cross-country skiers. *International Journal of Sports Medicine, 8*(2), 66–70.

Blum, R.H., et al. (1969). *Society and drugs.* San Francisco: Jossey-Bass.

Cohen, S. (1984). Drugs in the workplace. *Journal of Clinical Psychiatry, 45*(12), 4–8.

Cordova, V.F., & Banford, T.A. (1975). Experience in the identification of abuse drugs in urines collected under Treatment Alternatives to Street Crime. *Journal of Forensic Science, 20*(1), 58–70.

Council on Scientific Affairs. Issues in employee drug testing. (1987). *JAMA, 258*(15), 2089–2096.

Decker, W.J. (1977). Laboratory support of drug abuse control programs: An overview. *Clinical Toxicology, 10*(1), 23–35.

Goodman, A.G., Gilman, L.S., Rall, T.W., & Murad, F. (1985). *The pharmacological basis of therapeutics* (7th ed.). New York: Macmillan.

Haber, M.H. (1988). Pisse prophecy: A brief history of urinalysis. *Clinics in Laboratory Medicine 8*(3), 415–430.

Hall, R.C., Popkin, M.K., Devaul, R., & Stickney, S.K. (1977). The effect of unrecognized drug abuse on diagnosis and therapeutic outcome. *American Journal of Drug and Alcohol Abuse, 4,* 455–465.

Hall, R.C., Popkin, M.K., Stickney, S.K., & Gardner, E.R. (1978). Covert outpatient drug abuse. Incidence and therapist recognition. *Journal of Nervous and Mental Disease, 166,* 343–348.

Harvey, R. (1987, August 25). Pan Am Games: 1983 drug battle continues in '87. *Los Angeles Times*, Part III, pp. 1,11.

Hatton, C.K., & Catlin, D.H. (1987). Detection of androgenic anabolic steroids in urine. *Clinics in Laboratory Medicine, 7*(3), 655–668.

Hawks, R.L. (1986). Analytical methodology. In *Urine testing for drugs of abuse*. NIDA Research Monograph 73 (DHHS Publication No. ADM 84–1481). Washington, DC: Superintendent of Documents, U.S. Government Printing Office.

Hawks, R.L., & Chiang, C.N. (Eds.) (1986). *Urine testing for drugs of abuse*. NIDA Research Monograph 73 (DHHS Publication No. ADM 84–1481). Washington, DC: U.S. Government Printing Office.

Hoyt, D.W., Finnegan, R.E., Nee, T., Shults, T.F., & Butler, T.J. (1987). Drug testing in the workplace: Are methods legally defensible? A survey of experts, arbitrators, and testing laboratories. *JAMA, 258*, 504.

Jaffe, J.H. (1985). Drug addiction and drug abuse. In Goodman et al. (Eds.), *The pharmacological basis of therapeutics* (7th ed.). New York: Macmillan.

Kaistha, K.K. (1972). Drug abuse screening programs: Detection procedures, development costs, street-sample analysis, and field tests. *Journal of Pharmaceutical Sciences, 61*(5), 655–679.

Lederer, M. (1989). The role of chromatography and electrophoresis in biomedical sciences. *Journal of Chromatography, 488*, 5–24.

Los Angeles Times. (1986, October 29). Part I, p. 33.

Lundberg, G.D. (1972). Urine drug screening: Chemical McCarthyism. *New England Journal of Medicine, 287*(14), 723–724.

Lundberg, G.D. (1986). Mandatory unindicated urine drug screening: Still chemical McCarthyism. *JAMA, 256*(21), 3003–3005.

Mandatory guidelines for federal workplace drug testing programs: Final guidelines. (1988). (DHHS Publication.) Washington, DC: U.S. Government Printing Office.

Maugh, T.H. (1986, October 29). Navy viewed as setting drug testing standard. *Los Angeles Times*, Part I, p. 33.

Montagne, M, Pugh, C.B., & Fink, J.L. (1988). Testing for drug use: I. Analytical methods. *American Journal of Hospital Pharmacy, 45*, 1297–1305.

Morgan, J.P. (1984). Problems of mass urine screening for misused drugs. *Journal of Psychoactive Drugs, 16*(4), 305–317.

Murad, F., & Haynes, Jr., R.C. (1985). Adenohypophyseal hormones and related substances. In Goodman et al. (Eds.), *The pharmacological basis of therapeutics* (7th ed.). New York: Macmillan.

Musto, D.F. (1973). *The American disease*. New Haven, CT: Yale University Press.

National Commission on Marihuana and Drug Abuse (1973). *Drug use in America: Problem in perspective* (2nd report). Washington, DC: U.S. Government Printing Office.

National Institute on Drug Abuse (1982). *National household survey on drug abuse, 1982*. Rockville, MD: NIDA.

Prevention and detection of drug taking ('doping') at the IX British Commonwealth Games (1971). *Scottish Medical Journal, 16*(8), 364–368.

Puffer, J.C. (1986). The use of drugs in swimming. *Clinical Sports Medicine, 5*(1), 77–89.

Richards, L.G. (Ed.) (1981). *Demographic trends and drug abuse, 1980–1995.* NIDA Research Monograph 35. (DHHS Publication No. ADM 81–600065). Washington, DC: U.S. Government Printing Office.

Richardson, P., & Morein, M.J. (1979). Urine screening of arrestees as a source of drug abuse indicator data. *American Journal of Drug and Alcohol Abuse, 6*(4), 501–509.

Sohn, D. (1972). Drug screening—fact of life for the nineteen seventies. *Industrial Medicine, 41*(6), 18–21.

Sohn, D., Sohn, S., & Scott, L. (1970). Drug screening in industrial nursing. *Occupational Health Nursing, 18*(8), 7–10.

Sohn, D., & Simon, J. (1972). Rapid identification of psychopharmacologic agents in cases of drug abuse. *Clinical Chemistry, 18*(5), 405–409.

Swinyard, E.A. (1985). Principles of prescription order writing and patient compliance instruction. In Goodman et al. (Eds.), *The pharmacological basis of therapeutics* (7th ed.). New York: Macmillan.

West, L.J., & Cohen, S. (1985). Provisions for dependency disorders. In W.W. Holland, R. Detels, & G. Knox (Eds.), *Oxford textbook of public health* (Vol. 2). New York: Oxford University Press.

Winick, C. (1973). Some reasons for the increase in drug dependence among middle class youths. In H. Silverstein (Ed.), *Sociology of youth.* New York: Macmillan.

NOTES

1. For more comprehensive accounts of the history of drugs and their use, the reader is referred to *Society and Drugs* by Blum et al. (1969), *The American Disease* by Musto (1973), and to chapters on drug addiction by Jaffe and on individual drugs in *The Pharmacological Basis of Therapeutics,* edited by Goodman, Gilman, Rall, and Murad (1985).

2. *Drug Testing in Major U.S. Corporations: A Survey of the Fortune 500* (Raleigh, NC: Noel Dunivant and Associates, 1985).

2

The Politics of Drug Testing

J. MICHAEL WALSH AND JEANNE G. TRUMBLE

"True it is that politics makes strange bedfellows," wrote Charles Dudley Warner more than a century ago, and we are reminded of this adage as we look at the odd assortment of bedfellows that have shaped the current politics of drug testing.

In addition to the usual players—lawyers and politicians—the drug-testing roster includes pathologists, forensic toxicologists, civil libertarians, pharmaceutical manufacturers, laboratory associations, employee unions, security and law enforcement personnel, social and health service providers, victims groups, and assorted lobbyists for all the above who relentlessly bring political pressure to ensure that the rights, interests, and paychecks of their respective constituencies will be protected.

Drug abuse is a complicated social phenomenon. Over the last twenty years there has been a significant increase in the impact of drug abuse on the daily life of the average American. One cannot pick up a newspaper or watch a television newscast without being reminded of the tragic consequences of drug abuse. Drug-related crime, disease, accidents, injuries, deaths, and associated sordid details have become daily reminders of the limited effectiveness of supply-reduction efforts to reduce drug abuse.

There is, of late, a hue and cry from all segments of society to develop a change in focus and to concentrate efforts on reducing the demand for drugs. At this writing, however, the dollars available for the "war against drugs" on the supply (law enforcement) side significantly outstrip demand-side dollars (treatment, prevention, and education). Furthermore, the relationships between individual involvement in drug use, even for casual or recreational use, and the concomitant economic and health costs, as well as the assault on the moral fabric of American society, are only beginning to be recognized.

Recently the Reagan and Bush administrations have argued that the key

The opinions expressed herein are the views of the authors and do not necessarily reflect the official position of the National Institute on Drug Abuse or any other part of the U.S. Department of Health and Human Services.

to reducing the demand for drugs is to hold the individual drug user responsible for his or her behavior—to develop societal contingencies that censure and penalize the individual user with stiff sanctions (e.g., seizing assets or withholding the opportunity for employment). The environment in which this technique has been most effectively used is in the American workplace. Beginning with the military experience in the early 1980s, workplace programs have been developed to send a simple and direct message that drug use by employees will not be tolerated. Clearly, one of the key elements of such policies has been the use of drug-detection technology to identify drug users.

Even though drug detection by urinalysis is not a new technique (as is detailed historically in Chapter 1), drug testing has clearly become an issue in the 1980s. The Department of Defense (DOD) utilized urinalysis in the late 1960s and early 1970s to screen military personnel returning from Vietnam, and law enforcement officers and drug-treatment programs have used drug testing for many years. It was not until 1980, however, that new technology became available that provided a reliable and inexpensive assay for marijuana. The marketing of this new technology in 1981 occurred at roughly the same time as the DOD and the Congress (House Select Committee on Narcotics, 1981) independently reported the survey results of drug use by U.S. military personnel. The results of these two surveys indicated high rates of drug use by members of the military services and triggered considerable congressional scrutiny resulting in several acrimonious hearings in the fall of 1981 (Burt & Biegel, 1980). The unfortunate accident aboard the U.S. aircraft carrier *Nimitz* in May 1981, where drug use was discovered in the postmortem of the dead crew members, served also to fuel the fire that was smoldering in the Congress. The juxtaposition of these events—the availability of new drug-testing technology and congressional demands for the Defense Department to "do something" about the military drug problem—was pivotal in the justification for widespread application of drug-testing technology. In February 1982, the U.S. Navy was the first military branch to launch worldwide initiatives that included an on-site drug-testing capability on virtually every ship in the fleet.

The rationale for the use of drug testing has evolved considerably since 1981. The basic philosophy of why to test and what to do with the results of testing has changed dramatically during this time. Initially, the rationale for testing was a negative, punitive concept where the basic purpose was to identify drug users and dismiss them without addressing the problem. From about 1985 to the present, a more positive "helping-hand" philosophy has evolved. The basic purpose of today's model policy is to get substance-abusing employees into drug treatment, afford the opportunity to get help, and get the individual back on the job.

Despite the positive progress, the utilization of drug testing to make employment decisions generates an emotional, gut-level response from both labor and management. Before going into the details of the evolution of today's drug-testing politics and policies, it is important to be familiar with the basic issues with which management and labor have been struggling.

BASIC ISSUES: PROS AND CONS

The question of whether or not to utilize drug-testing technology evokes a complex array of moral, social, ethical, medical, scientific, and legal dilemmas for many Americans. Although most citizens do not condone drug abuse, their concerns about the erosion of civil liberties (similar to computer intrusions into privacy, the requiring of three kinds of identification to cash a check, metal detectors at airports, etc.) generate feelings of uncertainty as to whether the end justifies the means. Charles Krauthammer, a noted political analyst for *The Washington Post,* provides a good example of this ethical conflict. In August 1985, Krauthammer chided those in power, writing that "drug abuse has been elevated to the status of disease . . . which assures the victim that he is not to blame. The medical model—the user as victim—makes for more than bad pedagogy. It makes for bad policy." Krauthammer urged that we must do whatever is necessary to hold individuals responsible for their drug use. Subsequently, in April 1986, in the same paper, he wrote that the invasion of privacy required by drug testing goes too far: "If we are ever going to get a handle on the drug problem, it is going to have to be from the demand side. . . . Urine testing—I admit—is the most promising—indeed the only remaining—means of drug-enforcement. But its price is very high . . . choose liberty instead" (Krauthammer, 1986).

Many Americans view the drug-testing process (i.e., collection of urine) as degrading and dehumanizing. Government employees, employee unions, and civil libertarians argue strongly that drug testing is an invasion of privacy, that it constitutes an illegal search and seizure (i.e., of body fluids) and, therefore, violates individual rights guaranteed by the Constitution. In general, the constitutional protections apply only to testing conducted by the government (federal, state, and local). Government-mandated drug testing of private-sector employees—for example, in the federally regulated transportation and nuclear power industries—must also pass constitutional muster. Although several of these constitutional questions are currently before the Supreme Court, many may not be resolved by the current cases and will likely continue to be the subject of litigation for some time to come. This legal uncertainty, of whether testing will be upheld and programs go forward, or whether testing will be found unconstitutional and therefore go away, has created a great deal of confusion for policymakers as well as for employees and unions.

Medical and scientific questions about the accuracy and reliability of drug testing are continually raised by those who oppose testing. Concerns have been voiced that many laboratories currently engaged in offering drug-testing services do not have the expertise or capability to perform the assays required. In addition, many employers may be using inappropriate technology and falsely accusing employees of drug use. Congressional support for these concerns has been manifested by the passage of legislation (P.L. 100-71 sec. 503, July 11, 1987) that requires stringent technical and scientific procedures for federal workplace drug-testing programs, as well as standards for the certification of laboratories engaged in drug testing for federal agencies. Similar legislation has been introduced in both the U.S. Senate and House of Representatives, which would require such standards and lab certification for the private sector.

In response to concerns about the accuracy and reliability of drug testing, the U.S. Department of Health and Human Services (HHS) has issued "Mandatory Guidelines for Federal Workplace Drug Testing Programs" (1988). These guidelines are mandatory for federal programs and have rapidly become the gold standard for private-sector programs as well. The rigor of the federal standards has virtually dispensed with concerns regarding accuracy and reliability. The issue of the quality of laboratories has also been addressed by the HHS through the establishment of a National Laboratory Certification Program. The College of American Pathologists has also established a "Forensic Urine Drug Testing" certification program making "certified" labs available in virtually every state in the nation. The use of a "certified lab" has become the standard by which programs are being measured.

The American Civil Liberties Union (ACLU) has been among the most vocal organizations actively lobbying against drug testing. In addition to constitutional issues, a major concern about drug-testing programs has been the potential for abuse by managers and supervisors to discriminate and harass employees. The ACLU has made drug testing its number-one legislative initiative, and it is lobbying lawmakers in each of the fifty states to initiate legislation that would restrict or prohibit the use of drug testing. The focus of the ACLU argument is that a positive urinalysis does not prove intoxication, nor impairment of performance, and therefore cannot be used to draw a connection between drug use and work performance. The ACLU further argues that the testing of employees without cause (i.e., individualized reasonable suspicion of drug use) is unconstitutional.

On the pro side of drug testing, many employers feel a moral obligation to do all they can to achieve a drug-free workplace. In general, employers have wrestled with competing objectives and values to develop substance-abuse policies that fulfill several obligations. Employers have corporate responsibilities to (1) provide a healthy and safe workplace for all employees, (2) provide the best service/product to the customer, and (3) protect shareholders from losses due to drug abuse. On the other side of the equation, employers have obligations to their workers: (1) to respect the individual rights and civil liberties of their loyal and trustworthy employees (who for the most part are not involved with drugs); (2) to provide for reasonable expectations of privacy and confidentiality; and (3) to advise employees of the drug policy and the consequences of policy violation. This is an exceedingly difficult balancing act, and the balance will shift depending on the individual work site and the nature of the particular job.

To those who support vigorous use of testing, the facts are clear: the United States has a serious drug-abuse problem that threatens the health, welfare, and economy of the nation. The 1988 Household Survey on Drug Abuse conducted by the National Institute on Drug Abuse indicated that 28 million Americans (14 percent of the entire U.S. population over the age of twelve) had used an illicit substance within the last year. Moreover, drug testing has been shown to be effective in reducing substance abuse in the work force, reducing accidents and absenteeism, lowering health benefit utilization, and increasing productivity. And major employers (including the Department of Defense) report that drug testing is the cornerstone to an effective substance-abuse program. The U.S. Department of Labor (1989) has estimated that 20 percent of the private-sector labor force works in an establishment that has a drug-testing policy.

POLITICS IN THE 1980s

How has this political climate evolved? We will attempt to describe how the competing forces, interacting objectives, political considerations, technological advances, and serendipitous events that have occurred each year since 1981 have shaped the current politics of drug testing. After much deliberation as to the best way to organize the data, we have come to the conclusion that a chronological presentation of the facts, integrating public and private-sector initiatives, legislative actions, union activities, and significant media-related events, would allow the reader the greatest understanding of the process. Therefore, we begin the details of this decade-long chronicle with the germane happenings of 1981.

1981: Congress and the Military

Activities in 1981 focused mainly on the congressional assessment of the scope of the drug problem in the military services. The 1980 *Worldwide Survey* (Burt & Biegel, 1980) indicated that 26 percent of all military personnel had used marijuana in the thirty days prior to being surveyed. Ten percent reported the use of more than one illicit drug, and 21 percent reported diminished work performance due to drug use. The congressional survey (conducted under the leadership of Congressmen Glenn English and Benjamin Gilman, 1981) revealed an even bleaker situation. More than 50 percent of Navy personnel admitted "weekly or more frequent" marijuana use, and 29 percent reported cocaine use. A shocking

42.3 percent of all personnel surveyed reported on-the-job use of drugs or alcohol during the thirty days prior to the survey. At a congressional hearing in September 1981, General Louiselle, Assistant Secretary of Defense for Health Affairs, was ordered by the House Select Committee on Narcotics to develop a plan to deal with the serious drug problem these surveys had documented. Although "Select" committees have no real legislative power, several members of the Select Committee on Narcotics were also members of the House Armed Forces Appropriations Committee. The message was clear—either the DOD move quickly to attack the drug problem or its fiscal year 1983 budget would surely suffer. Within weeks, DOD directives were drafted authorizing the use of drug testing, and plans were set to consider the vast logistical, legal, and technological issues involved in its implementation.

About the same time, the Syva Corporation was beginning to market a new enzyme-mediated immunoassay test (EMIT) for marijuana and other highly abused drugs, available in a portable kit and well suited to the military's worldwide operations. The availability of this technology at this particular time was opportune and the purchase of EMIT kits allowed the DOD to plan for a rapid expansion to its laboratory-based program.

1982: Beginning of Private Sector Involvement

As the U.S. Navy began a large-scale assault on drug abuse with the implementation of an ambitious drug-testing program in February 1982 under the leadership of Rear Admiral P. J. Mulloy (see Chapter 5), the National Institute on Drug Abuse (U.S. Department of Health and Human Services) received guarded inquiries (often from attorneys representing firms that wished to remain anonymous) regarding the use of drug-testing technology, its reliability and accuracy, and the legality of its use in the private sector.

Also in 1982, directors of the utility and transportation industries were quietly meeting to discuss problems regarding drug use in society and more specifically by employees in their own companies. A task force was developed under the auspices of the Edison Electric Institute representing the gas, electric, and nuclear power industries to coordinate and produce model substance-abuse policies and to provide guidance as to the appropriate use of drug-testing technology.

Similar efforts, although considerably less organized, were under way in the transportation industry. In October, during a discussion on alcohol and drug use in transportation held at the annual meeting of the National Safety Council, a representative of the Greyhound Corporation indicated that his company had begun regularly scheduled drug testing of bus drivers. An audible gasp arose from those assembled. During the coffee break that followed, lively discussions ensued, and it became clear that various companies were considering drug testing but wanted to move slowly and to first observe the military's experience. The announcement by Greyhound and subsequent reports of unacceptable rates of positive drug tests in its drivers and applicants brought considerable pressure on companies that provided service to the traveling public to implement testing programs.

1983: Public Awareness of Drugs at Work

By 1983, there was a dramatic increase in media attention to the scope of drug abuse in the American workplace. A National Transportation Safety Board report (1983) indicated that seven train accidents occurring between June 1982 and May 1983—with numerous fatalities and more than $17 million in property damage—involved alcohol or other drugs. In response, the Federal Railroad Administration began a rule-making process that would take almost two years and, ultimately, in 1985, would require reasonable suspicion, postaccident, and applicant testing for covered positions. The Research Triangle Institute released the results of a study designed to determine the economic cost of drug abuse to society; their figure was $25.8 billion in 1983 dollars (Harwood et al., 1984). The Navy reported testing 1.8 million urine samples this year.

On August 22, 1983, *Newsweek* ran an eight-page cover story on drugs in the workplace, describing for the average American the vivid details that justify their statement that "the use of illegal drugs on the job has become a crisis for American business." By the end of the year many companies were reporting the implementation of drug-testing programs. On December 5, 1983, a *U.S. News & World Report* article, "Getting Tough on Drugs," documented the efforts of numerous companies with aggressive anti-drug programs, which included drug testing, polygraph examination, locker searches, and drug-sniffing dogs, all of which resulted in the firing of employees and the denial of employment to applicants. The article contained the prediction that "within 5 years you'll have to be clean to get a job."

Accounts of lawsuits against companies with testing policies also began to be regularly reported in 1983. Initial legal strategies relied heavily on federal statutes protecting against handicap discrimination. Generally, where drug testing was struck down by the courts or in arbitration it was the result of a poorly run program. For example, litigation concerning the New York and Washington, D.C., police departments was lost because administrators could not positively identify the source of the tainted specimens (see *Newsweek*, 1983).

At the same time, unions were beginning to negotiate agreements that permitted the limited use of drug testing under specified circumstances. The International Brotherhood of Teamsters and the Amalgamated Transit Workers Union were among the first to begin discussions and contract negotiations involving drug testing.

In June 1983 a two-day closed meeting, co-sponsored by the United States Olympic Committee and Hahnemann University, was held with sports-medicine specialists, chemists, forensic toxicologists, and endocrinologists to discuss substance abuse in Olympic athletes, especially the use of steroids. Much of the discussion focused on the development of a drug-testing policy to eradicate drugs from the planned 1984 Olympics to be held in Los Angeles. These activities marked a beginning awareness and a focusing on drug use in all sports, both amateur and professional, and the beginning of the wide application of drug testing as a tool to limit the effects of drugs in sports.

In recapitulating the events of 1983, we must include a brief summary of the decision of the U.S. Court of Appeals for the Second Circuit in the case of *Borsari* vs. *Federal Aviation Administration*. Although this case did not involve drug testing, we believe the decision, which upheld the firing of an air traffic controller for off-duty sale of drugs, significantly influenced the utilization of drug testing in safety and security-sensitive workplaces. The appeals court found that, although there was no evidence that Mr. Borsari used drugs either on or off the job, and had an excellent performance record

> We are persuaded by the FAA's simple but seemingly uncontrovertible reliance on the incompatibility of drugs with successful air traffic control. The phrase "promote the efficiency-of-service" cannot be so limited as to require the Agency to wait for an on-the-job violation before dismissing an offending employee. Indeed, it has repeatedly been held that where an employee's misconduct is in conflict with the mission of the agency, *dismissal without proof of a direct effect on the individual's job performance is permissible* [emphasis added] under the "efficiency of the service" standard.

This decision set a precedent that established a link between off-duty drug involvement and performance of a safety-sensitive job.

1984: Wait and See

This year was notable for the "wait and see" attitude that many employers took regarding drug testing. It was clear from discussions with many major corporations that no one wanted to be out front on this issue. Many companies believed that to develop a drug policy and to initiate testing would foster the image that the company had a "drug problem." The public relations impact of a drug-testing program could be disastrous if the timing was not right. In addition, the complexities of policy development, the emerging scientific and technical issues, logistical problems, and the litigious nature of the beast made 1984 a good year to wait and see how and what the competition was doing. Most companies, however, did not sit idle in 1984. Rather, they used this interim to research the issues and draft policy and implementation plans.

As the year progressed the handwriting on the wall became clearer— drug testing was here to stay! On August 5, 1984, the *Baltimore Sun* ran the headline DRUG TESTING INCREASINGLY BECOMING STAN-

DARD PROCEDURE AT WORKPLACE. Shortly thereafter, the American Medical Association's *AMA NEWS* (September 7, 1984) reported that drug testing had increased because the state of the art of the tests had improved—making the tests cheaper to run and more accurate; and companies had learned that drug abusers could cost them money.

Naturally, the events of 1984 were not without controversy. Lawsuits and arbitration caseloads were mounting rapidly. Reports of laboratory errors in the massive Navy program again raised concerns that the application of this state-of-the-art technology might be premature. Accounts of alleged horror stories that employees were ordered to strip naked and provide specimens in view of other employees, that supervisors targeted troublemakers and union officials for testing, and that civil liberties and due process were tossed out the window were often repeated in the news of 1984.

1985: A Change in Philosophy

The events of 1985 were remarkable because, although drug testing had been progressively becoming part of the American workplace for more than three years, the American public only now began to wake up to that fact and become interested. Many large employers (GM, IBM, Mobil, Exxon, etc.) began to establish and implement testing programs; major professional organizations held national meetings and developed policy positions; and these activities brought about a nationwide philosophical discussion as to the "appropriateness" of drug testing. Political commentators, economists, and civil rights activists focused their attention on the issues, and their positions were voiced in editorials and op-ed pages of virtually every newspaper in the country. Within a matter of months there was a self-proclaimed "drug-testing expert" (e.g., Sam Donaldson to Carl Rowan) on every political talk show (e.g., "Meet the Press" to "Agronsky and Co."), and freelance writers were authoring simplistic explanations of the complicated technology. During the year a great deal of misinformation was generated by the media, which led to greater confusion and a polarization of employers and workers on the issues.

Early in the year, BIZNET, the cable network of the U.S. Chamber of Commerce, aired the first of a series of specials on "Drugs in the Workplace" in which drug testing was discussed at length. Dr. Richard Lesher, president of the organization, stated clearly, "My message is to business people. Let's seek that goal of a drug-free environment. . . . I think there's been too much emphasis on the rights of the users and not enough emphasis on the rights of the people working with and around them, and the rights of the corporation as well." Although the Chamber of Commerce did not openly support drug testing at this time, the implication was clear.

In April 1985 the DOD issued a directive authorizing the establishment of the Civilian Employee Drug Abuse Testing Program (DOD, April 8,

1985). The stated purpose of this program was to assist in determining fitness for appointment, assignment to, or retention in, a critical job by identifying drug abusers and notifying them of the availability of appropriate counseling, referral, rehabilitation, or other medical treatment. Also in April the *Journal of the American Medical Association* published an article entitled "Crisis in Drug Testing: Results of the CDC [Centers for Disease Control] Blind Study" (Hansen, Caudill, & Boone, 1985), which, although it had nothing to do with employee drug testing, reinvigorated both union and ACLU opposition. (It is interesting to note that during this period numerous myths sprouted regarding the accuracy and reliability of testing methods. Despite the fact that these myths have been repeatedly debunked, they persist with each new generation of opposition.)

Another key event in April was the annual meeting of the American Occupational Medical Association, which offered a special workshop on drugs in the workplace. The association membership is comprised largely of corporate medical personnel, and this workshop was attended by senior corporate medical officers of major corporations. The interest was so intense that a subsequent two-day meeting was scheduled for November under the auspices of the American Academy of Occupational Medicine.

In midsummer 1985, a side issue arose concerning the proposal to test schoolchildren for drugs. A small high school in New Jersey proposed that all students submit to mandatory testing. The validity of the student testing proposal was an emotionally charged issue that was immediately challenged and, by December, was ruled unconstitutional by the New Jersey courts. Another issue tangential to workplace drug testing, which nonetheless received much attention in the press, was that of testing college athletes. The relevance of student and athlete testing proposals to the issue at large was the fear of an ever-broadening use of this technology, providing fodder for the civil-libertarian arguments against testing.

By August 1985, media reports further highlighted the growing problem of substance abuse in the workplace. *The Wall Street Journal* (August 8, 1985) reported that, in response to growing awareness of substance-abuse problems, more and more companies were requiring employee drug tests. Reports indicated that 25 percent of Fortune 500 companies screen job applicants. Furthermore, the *Journal* quoted the *Executive Recruiter News,* a trade publication, which had reported that urinalysis was used in 8 percent of the searches performed by executive recruiters. The most eye-opening data came from a widely reported telephone poll conducted by the Cocaine National Helpline, run by a New Jersey hospital. Seventy-five percent of callers admitted to using illegal drugs on the job; 64 percent said the drugs impaired job performance; 44 percent admitted selling drugs to fellow employees; 18 percent admitted having a drug-related accident; and 18 percent said they had stolen from their employers to support their drug habit.

In September the New York Chamber of Commerce sponsored a conference on "Drugs in the Workplace" at which major New York corporations presented their policies to eager attendees. Three major meetings conducted almost back to back in early November demonstrated the intense interest in the drug/workplace/testing issues. Although not always evident from the program, the principal focus of discussion was drug testing. The Bureau of National Affairs conference in Washington drew nearly four hundred attendees from thirty-one states. A seminar entitled "Employee Drug Testing: A Dilemma" held by the American Academy of Occupational Medicine in Chicago, drew nearly five hundred representatives from nearly every major corporation in America. The American Academy for Psychoanalysis meeting in New York had an equally large attendance for its conference on drug abuse. It was clear from the tone and focus of these meetings that testing had caused great divisiveness among the medical community. Identifying substance abusers and firing them without treatment was anathema to the profession. The real dilemma was that, while management had made up its mind to go forward with testing policies, the corporate medical community was still struggling with ways in which to satisfy management and, at the same time, conduct programs in a manner consistent with the goals of the medical profession.

During the last two months of 1985 drug testing issues remained in the limelight. But there was a noticeable difference in the underlying philosophy of the corporate approach to the problem. Concern over corporate drug-testing policies had given way to the concept of comprehensive drug-free workplace policies.

1986: Issue Becomes "How" Not "If"

By early 1986, programs were being designed and implemented by major and mid-sized private-sector employers at an increasingly rapid pace. This implementation can be seen as occurring in waves, with the utility and transportation industries constituting the first wave and major financial institutions, investment firms, and banks following suit; these businesses were joined by corporations with less obvious safety and security-sensitive positions. Throughout the course of the year, pro-active rather than reactive planning became more frequent, with noticeably more rational and sensitive approaches being taken by employers. These actions were due in part to the vocal opposition of unions to the increasingly widespread use of drug testing, to a growing awareness of the mounting costs associated with drug use, and to management's recognition that the detection of drug users was only one step in exercising their responsibility.

Attempts to determine "what to do" once an employee had been identified as a drug user led to the expansion of the concept and definition of

the essential elements of a more comprehensive drug-free workplace program. Companies began to utilize their employee assistance programs and
other components of their human resource and medical departments to
identify drug-abuse treatment resources, to reevaluate their insurance
benefits, and to plan for the posttreatment reintegration of valued employees into their work force.

Concurrently, major trends were notable at the federal level to develop
a national response to the problem; namely, the release of the *Report of
the President's Commission on Organized Crime,* the issuance of Executive Order 12564, which mandated a drug-free federal workplace, and the
passage of the Anti-Drug Abuse Act of 1986. The untimely deaths of
prominent sports figures, including University of Maryland basketball
star Len Bias and Cleveland Brown safety Don Rogers, catapulted drug
abuse and the search for solutions to the forefront of the national agenda.
Professional sports organizations, state legislatures, the U.S. Chamber of
Commerce, national health associations, major national labor unions, the
American Civil Liberties Union, and the courts simultaneously increased
the amount of attention and resources devoted to the search for solutions.

An example of this evolution was the response to the cocaine overdose
death of a Capital Cities/ABC employee on company property in 1984.
The company initially reacted by proposing to use drug-sniffing dogs and
other patently punitive measures to identify employees who used drugs.
But due to the outraged response by employees, Capital Cities/ABC modified its approach and created an advisory committee of managers and
employees charged with developing a responsible and responsive policy
that would meet the needs of both the company and its employees. Capital Cities/ABC's final policy has been touted as a model.

Prior to 1986, often knowing of no other alternatives, many companies
instituted only drug-testing programs or other single-focus approaches
(locker searches, use of drug-sniffing dogs, etc.). The media routinely focused on reporting terminations of employment: Pennzoil fired eighty-
five workers in the course of one nine-month period; at a General Motors
plant in Dayton, Ohio, forty-nine employees were arrested and twenty-
nine were fired. For those occupations in which the performance of one's
job demanded drug-free performance at all times (e.g., pilots, those who
work with explosives, railroad employees, bus drivers, etc.), testing programs received less assault.

Outcomes of drug-testing initiatives began to be reported in 1986. For
example, in the first two years of its testing program, Southern Pacific
Railroad experienced a 72 percent drop in the number of accidents; on-
the-job injuries and sick days were also reduced. Incidents of widespread
firing, combined with the encouraging reports of reduced accidents, reduced absenteeism, and reduced health care utilization resulting from the
implementation of drug testing, accelerated the conflict between supporters and detractors of drug testing.

In early March the President's Commission on Organized Crime (March 1986) issued its final report. Among the more than fifty recommendations were the following:

> The President should direct the heads of all Federal agencies to formulate immediately clear policy statements, with implementing guidelines, including suitable drug testing programs, expressing the utter unacceptability of drug abuse by Federal employees. State and local governments and leaders in the private sector should support unequivocally a similar policy that any and all use of drugs is unacceptable. Government contracts should not be awarded to companies that fail to implement drug programs, including suitable drug testing.
>
> Government and private sector employers who do not already require drug testing of job applicants and current employees should consider the appropriateness of such a testing program.

Mr. Arthur Brill of the Commission was reported by *USA TODAY* (March 7, 1986) to have equated drug screening to taking vision tests before getting a driver's license. The American Federation of Government Employees loudly voiced Fourth Amendment concerns and stated its opposition to the "witch-hunt mentality." (*Washington Post,* March 14, 1986). Mr. Allan Adler of the ACLU expressed concern about the fallibility of the tests (Marcus & Engel, 1986). The U.S. Chamber of Commerce took the position that "The innocent have nothing to fear . . ." (*Washington Post,* Feb. 2, 1986, p. A14).

The simmering pot now began to boil. Most major newspapers, professional journals, business meetings, magazines, and the electronic media provided a forum for debate. An editorial in the *Washington Post* on March 14, 1986, referred to the drug-testing recommendations of the commission's report as a "crazy proposal." The *Post* did, however, note that drug testing with prior notification in certain categories of high-risk jobs is acceptable. Because the commission's report did not specifically address how testing was to be done, who would pay, and what would happen to employees who tested positive for drugs, the controversy raged over both the conceptual basis and specific implementation issues. An editorial in the *New York Times* in March 1986 described the negative reaction to the report by some members of Congress and the ACLU, but went on to say that the report "dramatizes the need for real answers to the real questions." The *Times* further stated that the limits of the law enforcement approach are clear; what else to do is not.

As the lead federal agency with national responsibility for addressing drug abuse in the nation, the National Institute on Drug Abuse (NIDA) convened what was to be called "a landmark" conference in March 1986. The conference was designed to discuss and achieve consensus on drug-testing issues. Scientists, attorneys, health and safety experts, corporate human resource and medical directors representing the Fortune 1000, and representatives of labor unions and the ACLU were invited to participate. Prior to the issuance of the *Report of the President's Commission on Organized Crime,* it appeared that reaching consensus would be extremely difficult; certain battle lines were firmly drawn with the unions and the ACLU being adamantly opposed to drug testing under any circumstances. However, the fortuitous release of the commission's report with its sweeping recommendations two days before the scheduled conference dramatically shifted the positions taken by attendees. Events and the passage of time had overtaken the posturing in the field; most attendees came prepared to enter into hard negotiations. The definition of the "acceptability" of testing had shifted. Prior to the release of the report, the position of the National Institute on Drug Abuse, which advocated testing for critical and sensitive positions, had been viewed as radical. Once the recommendation for the widespread testing of everyone employed in both the public and private sectors was posited by the commission, however, the NIDA stance became a reasonable accommodation. The conferees could then focus on prescribing the conditions under which testing would be conducted—conditions that would respect the individual rights and civil liberties of employees while meeting the needs of employers to maintain drug-free workplaces. After lengthy discussions, consensus was reached on the following:

- All individuals tested must be informed.
- All positive results on an initial screen must be confirmed through the use of alternate methodology.
- The confidentiality of test results must be assured.
- The use of urine drug testing must be accompanied by the opportunity for drug abuse treatment.
- Random screening for drug abuse under a well-defined program employing neutral criteria is also appropriate and legally defensible in certain circumstances.

The same shift in focus now became apparent in the media. Articles, interviews, and editorials began to discuss "how," not "if." *Time* magazine reporters had covered the NIDA consensus meeting and aptly summarized the national views on testing programs. Within a week, *Time* featured a cover story, "Drugs on the Job," which ran an unprecedented ten pages of the forty-four pages of news in the issue of March 17, 1986. At the same time, major employers who had programs in place for several years began to discuss their results, successes, and failures. J. Patrick Sanders, vice-president of Commonwealth Edison, reported a decrease in absenteeism, a slowing in the trend of increasing medical claims, and fewer on-the-job accidents. Although he stopped short of attributing this directly to his company's drug-testing program, he said, "It's got to be more than coincidental" (*Time,* March 17, 1986). There was an increasing recognition that carefully monitored and controlled drug testing could be an effective technique for identifying drug users and getting them into treatment, and that perhaps the most important effect was that of deterrence. That is, many employees would stop using drugs because they were afraid they would be caught and lose their job.

Some states considered legislation to restrict or regulate drug testing. For example, the Substance Abuse Testing Act of 1986 was introduced in the California legislature (March 1986) to establish safeguards to ensure the fairness and accuracy of substance abuse testing. This legislation was supported by the California Chamber of Commerce, the Brotherhood of Locomotive Engineers, and the Brotherhood of Railway and Airline Clerks.

Additionally, during hearings related to a bill before the Maryland legislature on drug testing, a representative of the Maryland ACLU stated that if an employer has a rehabilitation program, urinalysis could be performed (*National Law Journal*, 1986).

Public opinion polls conducted by *USA Today* in March 1986 and by the *New York Times*/CBS in August 1986 showed a parallel shift in public opinion as compared to earlier years. When randomly selected adults from across the United States were asked by *USA Today* whether they would object to being tested, 77 percent said no; 21 percent said yes; and 2 percent weren't sure. Of these same respondents, 62 percent supported and 29 percent opposed mandatory testing for federal workers and employees of government contractors; 43 percent supported drug testing in private firms, with 48 percent opposed. The *New York Times*/CBS Poll found that approximately three-fourths of full-time workers were willing to take a drug test; they did not see it as an unfair invasion of their privacy (Clymer, 1986). It must be noted that by this time the National Collegiate Athletic Association had introduced drug testing in all sports championships; the Federal Aviation Administration and the U.S. Customs Service were among the civilian federal agencies conducting tests; the U.S. Navy noted that the single most important factor in the reduction of drug use in the Navy was the drug-testing program; and approximately 26 percent of the Fortune 500 companies were screening applicants and employees.

By midyear 1986, it became clear that major presidential initiatives focusing on drugs in the workplace were taking shape, some of which were direct responses to the recommendations put forth by the President's Commission on Organized Crime. With regard to drug testing, multiple task forces were convened, composed of representatives of major federal agencies, notably the Department of Justice, the Office of Personnel Management, and the Department of Health and Human Services. Lengthy and intense sessions were devoted to hammering out the myriad of logistical details that needed to be in place to coordinate program development in more than 150 extremely diverse federal agencies. As attention became more intensely riveted on the mechanics of implementation, President Ronald Reagan issued Executive Order 12564, which mandated a drug-free federal workplace and clearly stated that the use of illegal drugs, whether on or off the job, was unacceptable for any federal employee (*Federal Register,* September 15, 1986).

Each agency was required to develop a plan with the following required components:

1. A statement of policy setting forth the agency's expectations regarding drug use and the action to be anticipated in response to identified drug use
2. Employee Assistance Programs, emphasizing high-level direction, education, counseling, referral to rehabilitation, and coordination with available community resources
3. Supervisory training to assist in identifying and addressing illegal drug use by agency employees
4. Provisions for self-referrals as well as supervisory referrals to treatment with maximum respect for individual confidentiality consistent with safety and security issues
5. Provision for identifying illegal drug users, including testing on a controlled and carefully monitored basis.

Although the private sector was increasingly implementing drug-free workplace programs, which included a testing component, considerable congressional debate took place regarding the advisability of drug testing for federal employees. Representative Pat Schroeder (D-Colo.), who headed the Subcommittee on Civil Service of the House Committee on Post Office and Civil Service, released a staff study in June 1986 attacking the reliability of testing and the constitutionality of random testing; the study questioned "whether it is appropriate for the Federal government to use its employees as the guinea pigs in the war against drugs" (Subcommittee on Civil Service, 1986).

The first legal battle of the federal initiative was the National Treasury Employees Union suit against the U.S. Customs Service (*NTEU* v. *von Raab*). U.S. District Court Judge Robert F. Collins (Eastern Louisiana) ruled that mandatory testing of certain employee-applicants of the U.S. Customs Service without individualized suspicion of drug use was unconstitutional under the Fourth, Fifth, Ninth, and Tenth Amendments. In his opinion, Judge Collins stated that

> this gross invasion of privacy constitutes a degrading procedure that so detracts from human dignity and self-respect that it "shocks the conscience" and offends this Court's sense of justice. . . . Customs workers do maintain a legitimate expectation of privacy in their urine until the decision is made to flush the urine down the toilet. The Customs Directive violates a legitimate expectation of privacy held by Customs workers (*NTEU* vs. *von Raab*).

On appeal, the Fifth Circuit reversed the decision of the lower court. Subsequently this case was appealed to the U.S. Supreme Court (see p. 44).

Among the first major professional organizations to take a formal stance, the American Occupational Medical Association (AOMA) released on July 25, 1986, "Ethical Guidelines on Drug Screening in the Workplace." These Guidelines dealt only with ethical issues and not with the more basic issues concerning the design and implementation of a drug-screening program. The AOMA policy states: "If carefully designed and carried out, employer-required programs for the screening of employees and applicants for drugs, including alcohol, can serve to protect and improve employee health and safety in an ethically acceptable manner" (American Occupational Medical Association, 1986).

As an example of Charles Dudley Warner's statement about politics making strange bedfellows, the National Organization for the Reform of Marijuana Laws (NORML) entered the fray. In September 1986, NORML filed a petition with the Food and Drug Administration requesting regulation of the commercial urine-testing industry, prohibition of the marketing of over-the-counter urine tests, institution of a quality-control program to ensure accurate testing, and sanctions against a specific commercial company for past testing errors (NORML, 1986). The Epilepsy Foundation of America went on record supporting regulation of the drug-testing industry; this was an issue of special significance to the foundation because of its association with drugs to control epilepsy. Among other concerns, the foundation wished to protect against false accusations of illegal drug use, the release of confidential medical information, and discrimination against those suffering from epilepsy (Epilepsy Foundation of America, 1986).

During this time of struggling with how to achieve drug-free workplaces as one step in ridding the nation of drugs, "crack" (a potent cocaine derivative) appeared on the scene. Heightened public awareness of the deadly effects of widespread cocaine and crack use created a political, economic, and social environment conducive to change. Private employers were more carefully designing and implementing their testing programs, and comprehensive programs were being developed where the threat of discharge was among many alternatives. Major corporations were designing their programs in relation to the specific needs of their unique work environment and work force, ensuring that the policy applied equally to *every* employee, including the boss. The courts and arbitrators seemed to agree, for the most part, that employees' civil rights do not extend to endangering the safety and welfare of others.

Early and serious involvement of unions greatly contributed to the likelihood of the development of a policy that protected both labor and management. The International Brotherhood of Teamsters was one of the first large and powerful unions to develop major programs, but within the unions, widely differing opinions were held (*Newsday Business,* 1986). Peter Bensinger, former administrator of the Drug Enforcement Administration (*Nation's Business,* 1986), postulated that union leaders viewed drug testing as a bargaining issue, but if members were to vote on drug testing, they would vote for it. The Oil, Chemical and Atomic Workers

Union, representing 1,500 workers at a Texas refinery, entered into an agreement with Amoco in which employees who tested positive would be sent for rehabilitation or suspended; they would then be subject to retest anytime over the next two years, and would be subject to dismissal were they to fail again. This agreement had been worked out between the Union and Amoco after the union had won a 1985 court order blocking a drug-testing program; the order was lifted when Amoco agreed to work on the compromise (*Newsday Business,* 1986).

The strong economy that the country enjoyed in 1986 produced a heavy demand for qualified employees. The large applicant pool combined with a significant number of new hires was another major factor that allowed employers to implement pre-employment urine drug-testing programs. A 1986 Employment Management Association (EMA) national survey of human resource professionals showed that approximately 29 percent of respondents reported that their companies had pre-employment alcohol/drug testing programs and approximately 21 percent reported having employee testing programs. EMA also reported that prior to 1984 only 3 percent of employers tested either group (Dickey, 1987). Since applicants for jobs are often not viewed as having the same rights as employees, pre-employment testing programs avoided much of the controversy created by the testing of current employees.

1987: Era of Refinement

The year 1986 can be viewed as pivotal in the movement away from simple "drug testing" programs. The reasonableness and appropriateness for employers to implement substance-abuse programs was no longer the issue. Rather, the question became how such programs could be conducted fairly and effectively, and 1987 began the era of refinement and incorporation of testing within larger and more comprehensive substance-abuse programs. Recognizing that drug testing was a reality and desiring to exercise some control, well-established and prestigious professional groups began to focus on drug-testing issues. Major meetings of the American Medical Association, the American Bar Association, and other organizations all featured a section on employee drug testing. Formal position statements were developed and solidified. Even smaller specialized groups (e.g., industrial hygienists) began to hold formal discussions regarding substance-abuse policy. Meanwhile, the federal program became much more clearly defined with the passage of Public Law 100-71 and the issuance of "Mandatory Guidelines for Federal Workplace Drug Testing Programs," which included standards for the certification of laboratories.

Not unexpectedly, the marketplace demonstrated aggressive pursuit of profits: attorneys saw potential gain from a never-ending series of lawsuits; laboratories anticipated increased demand for their services; private consultants sold their knowledge and materials to companies searching for solutions; and inventors of testing technologies applied their creativity to develop novel products. With the drug-testing field growing an estimated 10 percent a year, profit motives provided stiff competition to humanitarian concerns.

Meanwhile, in the nation's corporate boardrooms, the operating philosophy became that *if* the company should choose to institute drug testing as part of the response to drug problems, it should be done *right*—that is, using proper procedures, applying proper scientific and health principles, and in a manner demonstrating utmost regard for the rights and expectations of employees, employers, and the public.

Early in January 1987, a Conrail train filled with college students and others returning home after the Christmas holidays crashed in Chase, Maryland, killing sixteen passengers, injuring 174, and causing millions of dollars in property damage. Urine specimens collected under the authority of the Federal Railroad Administration's drug regulations revealed that the Conrail engineer and brakeman had been smoking marijuana. On January 21, 1987, the U.S. Department of Transportation proposed rigorous drug-testing programs requiring pre-employment, post-accident, and random testing of airline pilots, railroad workers, air traffic controllers, and other employees in safety-related positions. Although these regulations had been under consideration for a long period of time, public acceptability appeared to have been greatly enhanced by their memory of the recent Conrail accident. In January 1987, The *Washington Post* quoted W. Graham Claytor, president and chairman of the board of the federally owned Amtrak rail system, expressing his belief that random drug testing and testing as part of annually required physical examinations were essential to ensuring public safety (Lancaster, 1987). The 1985 Federal Railroad Administration rule limiting testing in the railroad industry to post-accident and reasonable suspicion circumstances did not appear to protect the public sufficiently, allowing for detection only after an accident occurred.

In the spring of 1987, according to an update of state and local legislative proposals regarding drug testing prepared by the Equal Employment Advisory Council, "drug testing laws had been enacted in Iowa, Minnesota, Montana, Utah, and Vermont and nearly thirty other states were considering, or had considered the issue. Many of the bills create specific rights for employees, or place restrictions on testing by employers. . . . New laws in Iowa, Minnesota, Montana and Vermont largely restrict employer testing without probable cause or reasonable suspicion. Others, such as the law enacted in Utah, would grant employers considerable flexibility in administering drug tests, and a proposed Colorado bill would grant a state tax credit to employers who put employees through an assistance program" (Equal Employment Advisory Council, 1987).

At the federal level, except for the Department of Defense, the Federal Aviation Administration, and the U.S. Customs Service, very few agencies were actually engaged in drug testing in 1987. On February 19, 1987, a press conference was held at the Department of Health and Human

Services to announce issuance of the "Mandatory Guidelines for Federal Workplace Drug Testing Programs," required by the president's Executive Order. With HHS Secretary Otis R. Bowen, Attorney General Edwin Meese, and Office of Personnel Management Director Constance Horner presiding, issuance of the Mandatory Guidelines reawakened the debate over many of the issues pertaining to whether or not testing was a legitimate approach to solving drug problems. Many new players entered the game (e.g., congressional members from Maryland, Virginia, and the District of Columbia, locales with huge federal employee constituencies) who had not participated in the early years of discussions and decisions. The government unions (including the American Federation of Government Employees, National Treasury Employees Union, National Association of Government Employees) and the media started another furor, much of it limited to inside the Beltway, which rings Washington, D.C.

About this time (spring 1987), as the agencies began formulating implementation plans, Congressman Steny Hoyer (D-Md.), member of the House Appropriations Committee, tendered a bill to prohibit the expenditure of appropriated monies by federal agencies for drug testing. Before the Hoyer bill received committee attention, the Reagan administration worked out a compromise with a bipartisan group representing both sides of Capitol Hill. In early June, an extraordinary meeting took place among the Attorney General, the Secretary of Transportation, the Secretary of Health and Human Services, and the Directors of the Office of Management and Budget, and the Office of Personnel Management (all representing the Reagan administration) and Senators Barbara Mikulski, Dennis DeConcini, and Pete Domenici and Congressman Hoyer (representing the Congress). The outcome of this high-stakes meeting was passage of Section 503, Title V, Public Law 100-71, which permitted the administration to proceed with programs to test federal employees provided a number of parameters were met.

Public Law 100-71 specified that any federal employee who was the subject of a drug test shall, upon written request, have access to any records relating to the test and that results of a drug test may not be disclosed without prior written consent of the employee unless the disclosure would be to the employee's medical review officer, the administrator of the Employee Assistance Program (EAP) or to agency officials having authority to take adverse personnel action. One of the most significant aspects of P.L. 100-71 was the requirement that the U.S. Department of Health and Human Services publish new mandatory guidelines for federal drug-testing programs that (1) establish comprehensive standards for all aspects of laboratory drug testing and laboratory procedures; (2) specify the drugs for which federal employees may be tested; and (3) establish appropriate standards and procedures for periodic review of laboratories and criteria for certification and revocation of certification of laboratories to perform drug testing in carrying out Executive Order 12564. The bill furthermore required the Secretary of Health and Human Services to review and certify to the Congress that all federal agency plans meet applicable provisions of law and the Executive Order and that *none* of the major agencies could start *until all* were certified (P.L. 100-71).

Initially it seemed that fulfilling the requirements of Section 503 of P.L. 100-71 was an impossible task. Getting more than 150 federal agencies to toe the mark and develop plans that met the legislation's provision of "uniformity and consistency" appeared to be an unattainable goal. Many felt that the Congress had made a brilliant move allowing the bureaucracy to kill the program by its own weight—strangling in the complexities imposed by P.L. 100-71. Federal activities for the remainder of 1987 were concentrated on getting the largest federal agencies to finalize their plans in a certifiable manner, and refining the technical and scientific standards for the drug-testing component.

1988: Federal Program Implementation

With the parameters of the federal program clearly defined, federal agencies were developing implementation strategies for their drug-free workplace programs awaiting only final publication of the technical and scientific guidelines for the testing portion. The "Mandatory Guidelines for Federal Workplace Drug Testing Programs" were published in the *Federal Register* on April 11, 1988, setting the stage for full program implementation. The Mandatory Guidelines set out the scientific and technical procedures for testing and the standards for laboratories seeking the certification required to conduct drug tests for federal employees. In the interests of protecting employees and ensuring accuracy and reliability of the testing procedures, these standards were extremely rigorous. As a result, strong opposition to the standards and particularly to the certification program was mounted by those who predicted negative financial impact if they failed to meet the "gold standard" that had been established.

The controversy was further fueled with discussion regarding the imposition of the federal employee program (as described in Executive Order 12564, P.L. 100-71 and the Mandatory Guidelines) onto federal contractors, grantees, and the private sector. The issuance of regulations for defense contractors (Department of Defense) and discussions among members of the Congress to require that all federal contractors and grantees comply with the federal program created panic among many of the smaller nondefense contractors as well as grantee institutions in the academic community, which saw a threat to academic freedom. Rumors were rampant, and some of the basic issues about testing were again raised by an entirely different segment of the work force.

In October 1988, the Drug Free Workplace Act (P.L. 100-690) was passed by the Congress. The act required all federal contractors with contracts in excess of $25,000 and federal grant recipients (of any amount) to have a written policy regarding workplace substance abuse, to establish a drug awareness program, and to report instances of employee's workplace drug-related convictions. Although the law did not require drug testing, it provided the impetus to many employers who had been contemplating a testing program.

The first tier of the forty-two largest federal agencies (representing a work force in excess of 2 million employees) had their plans certified by the head of the Department of Health and Human Services to the U.S. Congress on April 27, 1988. As each agency issued implementation notices to employees, federal employee unions loudly opposed the program and litigation increased dramatically.

In the fall, the U.S. Supreme Court announced it would hear two drug-testing cases: the U.S. Customs Service case (*NTEU* vs. *von Raab*) and a case brought against the Secretary of Transportation (*RLEA* vs. *Burnley*) involving post-accident testing in the railroad industry. Although there were those federal agencies who saw pending litigation as a convenient reason to delay implementation, by the end of 1988 most components of the federal program were well on their way to full implementation.

A midyear editorial in the *New York Times* (July 12, 1988) summed up the significant progress of drug-policy development:

> Law and public perceptions have come a long way since the Plainfield, N.J., fire department raided its own fire station two years ago, roused sleeping firefighters and demanded urine samples on the spot. The Reagan program addresses the need for fair warning to employees and job applicants, dignified yet reliable collection of samples, safeguards against false results and considerate behavior toward users willing to accept help.

1989: Supreme Ct. Upholds Testing

The expectations of the anti-drug-testing forces that Democratic presidential candidate Michael Dukakis would win the presidency and save the country from the "evils of drug testing" were dashed by the election of George Bush. Bush throughout his election campaign spoke strongly in favor of the use of drug testing as an essential tool in the fight against drug abuse.

It appeared at the outset of 1989 that the Reagan initiatives on drug testing would continue without suffering through the transition of a new administration. However, the anti-drug act of 1988 required the new president to appoint a "drug czar" and to establish a new Office of National Drug Control Policy (ONDCP) within the Executive Office of the President to coordinate all federal agency drug activities and initiatives. This new office was established quickly. Dr. William Bennett (former Secretary of Education in the Reagan administration) was confirmed as the director of ONDCP by the Senate in March, and the new "National Drug Control Strategy" was developed and submitted to the Congress in record time (September 5, 1989). However, during this transition (from the election in November 1988 to September 1989) an uncertainty was felt throughout the federal sector. Questions were raised as to whether President Bush fully supported employee drug testing and whether his "drug czar" Dr. Bennett agreed. Many programs marked time during this year-long period, waiting for a "clear sign" from the new president that the federal drug-free workplace programs, including drug testing, were to go forward.

The year began with numerous lawsuits being filed opposing federal agency programs. Even employees of the Office of Management and Budget in the president's own Executive Office sued to block mandatory drug tests (*Hartness* vs. *Bush*). In January, U.S. District Court Judge Harold Greene granted an injunction blocking the random testing component of the Department of the Interior's drug-free workplace program, calling the department's program "a bureaucracy run amok." Most case decisions at the federal, district, and circuit court of appeals, however, were delayed awaiting direction from the Supreme Court, which had agreed in October 1988 to hear arguments on two drug-testing cases (*NTEU* vs. *von Raab, RLEA* vs. *Burnley*).[1]

On March 21, 1989, the U.S. Supreme Court handed down its first decisions on testing for drug abuse in the workplace. In *RLEA* vs. *Skinner* the Court upheld the Federal Railroad Administration's regulation authorizing mandatory drug testing without individualized suspicion of drug use for certain rail employees following major train accidents. The High Court found that blood and urine tests for railroad workers involved in accidents were constitutional and did not violate privacy rights even when there was no evidence in advance of individual drug or alcohol abuse. In *NTEU* vs. *von Raab*, the Supreme Court upheld the constitutionality of urine drug tests for U.S. Customs Service employees seeking drug-enforcement jobs. In writing for the majority in both cases, Justice Anthony Kennedy agreed that both blood and urinalysis tests are "searches" under the Fourth Amendment; however, such testing constituted "reasonable" search under the Fourth Amendment since "the government interest in testing without a showing of individualized suspicion is compelling."

One of the important outcomes of the two Supreme Court decisions was the discussion of the procedural aspects of drug testing. In *RLEA* vs. *Skinner* the Court found "no reason for doubting the agency's conclusion that the tests at issue are accurate in the overwhelming majority of cases." The Court therefore rejected the Ninth Circuit's concerns over the reliability of testing. In *NTEU* vs. *von Raab* the Court, in balancing the needs of the government against the intrusion of individual privacy, concluded that the procedures provided for under the Mandatory Guidelines, 53 *F. Reg.* 11970 (11 April 1988), "significantly minimize the intru-

---

1. When Samuel Skinner succeeded James Burnley as Secretary of Transportation the case was renamed *RLEA* vs. *Skinner.*

siveness of the Service's drug screening program." As a result of these two decisions, issues related to the accuracy and reliability of the testing technology are generally no longer raised in litigation.

Although neither of these initial cases involved "random testing," the Supreme Court subsequently has denied *certiorari* in several instances, thus allowing to stand lower court decisions finding "random testing" constitutional (*Utility Workers* vs. *So. Cal. Edison Co.*, No. 88-1180 (U.S. 3/20/89); *Policeman's Benevolent Assn. of New Jersey* vs. *Washington Township*, No. 88-706). By midyear there were nearly fifty suits filed in federal courts around the country. The majority of case decisions supported the use of testing, but each case further defined the conditions under which testing was considered to be appropriate.

Various polls in 1989 continued to indicate an ever-increasing growth in employee drug testing and public support for the use of testing. Early in the year the Bureau of Labor Statistics (BLS) issued a report of a nationally representative survey of some 7,500 private-sector business establishments with regard to drug testing and EAP programs (Department of Labor, 1989). Probably the most significant finding of the BLS survey was that 20 percent of the private-sector work force (estimated to be 17 million workers out of a total private-sector [nonagricultural] work force of 85 million) worked in an establishment with a drug-testing program. Overall, 3.2 percent of all businesses surveyed had a testing program. This ranged from less than 1 percent doing testing in very small businesses (fewer than ten employees) to 60 percent in large companies (more than 5,000 employees). Twelve percent of approximately 4 million job applicants tested positive in the year prior to the survey. Nearly 9 percent of 1 million in-service employees tested positive in this same period.

The California Poll, conducted by the Fields Institute in April 1989, indicated that eight out of ten Californians said they would submit to a random drug test, and that an overwhelming majority want people tested who hold "sensitive" jobs such as pilots, train engineers, police officers, firefighters, and bus drivers. This study was identical to one conducted two years previously, and in practically every category the new poll showed greater acceptance of random drug testing (see Table 2.1) (*Sacramento Bee*, 1989). Not surprisingly, acceptance of testing varied directly as a function of political conservatism, with 93 percent of the "conservatives" indicating a willingness to be tested, 84 percent of the "moderates," and 65 percent of the "liberals."

Further support for the legitimacy of drug testing is evident in the increasing political pressure to establish federal legislation to impose standards for employee drug testing—a trend first noted in the mid-1980s. Congressmen John Dingell (D-Mich.) and Thomas J. Bliley (R-Va.) introduced a bill to establish a federal standard for test procedures and require the use of certified laboratories for *all* employee drug testing conducted

TABLE 2.1   The California Poll

People Interviewed	1989	1987
Proportion Favoring Random Drug Testing in Professions		
Airline pilots	92%	87%
Bus drivers, train engineers, and ship captains	92	86
Police, firefighters	89	85
State-elected officials	78	68
Public schoolteachers	78	65
Professional athletes	75	63
College athletes	73	65
Proportion Willing to Submit to Random Drug Testing		
STATEWIDE	83%	77%
Men	80	73
Women	85	80
Conservatives	93	85
Moderates	84	80
Liberals	65	57
18–29 years of age	80	68
30–39 years of age	69	69
40–49 years of age	81	78
50–59 years of age	93	85
60 years or older	94	91

in the United States. Similar legislation was introduced in the Senate by Senators Orrin Hatch (R-Utah) and David Boren (D-Ok.). There appears to be support from both business and labor on these initiatives. Business is supportive of a preemptive federal statute that would eliminate the various state laws that have been enacted within the last two to three years. Because these state statutes vary considerably, businesses that have multistate operations must have a different policy for each state. Business appears ready to support federal legislation if such legislation will allow sufficient flexibility to employers. Labor is supportive of federal legislation that would provide protections for employees, guarantee due process, and place required procedural standards for collection and analysis of urine specimens. If consensus can be achieved between business and labor on the details of procedures and analysis, it seems likely that federal legislation on employee drug testing will soon be enacted.

As in 1987, similar activities were ongoing at the state level; by year's end, at least sixteen states and several local jurisdictions had some type of state and local drug-testing requirements, many of which include testing of state employees (National Foundation for the Study of Employment Policy, 1989).

SUMMARY

As evident as early as 1987, employee drug testing is here to stay. Much has happened during the last ten years, but the battle on drug testing is not over, and the war on drugs has not been won. Despite considerable efforts to develop more fair, equitable, and comprehensive policies, policies that use testing primarily as a tool for the early identification of those who need help, the conflict over testing rages on.

In our view, legal decisions on drug testing have been influenced to a great extent by the political climate of the day. Inevitably, legal decisions take on a life of their own and ultimately determine the course of future political events. This cycle has manifested itself repeatedly throughout the course of history in the United States (e.g., abortion and civil rights), and we see no reason that the political course of drug testing will be any different. Although the acceptability of drug testing appears to be increasing, there will continue to be grievances and lawsuits filed. And there will continue to be those who cling to the belief that some court decision will strike down drug testing on constitutional or other legal grounds.

We firmly believe that, realistically, no single action, in and of itself, will determine the course of future events. In the short term, however, the effects of specific incidents (e.g., the release of data supporting the beneficial outcomes of a testing program, or an adverse legal decision striking down a testing program) will cause emotions to run high and serve only to drive the wedge even further between the two sides in this continually unfolding drama.

REFERENCES

American Medical Association. (1984, September 7). *AMA News.*

American Occupational Medical Association. (1986, July 25). *Ethical guidelines on drug screening in the workplace.*

Burt, M.R., & Biegel, M.M. (1980). *Worldwide survey of nonmedical drug use and alcohol among military personnel,* Bethesda, MD: Burt Associates, Inc.

Business' war on drug abuse. (1986, October). *Nation's Business,* pp. 18–26.

California State Legislature, Substance Abuse Testing Act of 1986 (AB 4242). (1986, March).

Clymer, A. (1986, September 2). Public found ready to sacrifice in drug fight. *The New York Times,* p. A1.

Dickey, E.P. (1987, Winter). EMA survey shows extent of alcohol/drug testing in the workplace. *The EMA Journal.*

Department of Defense. (1988, September 28). Federal acquisition regulation supplement, drug-free workplace, 48 CFR, parts 223 and 252.

Department of Defense Directive. (1985, April 8). Subject: DOD Civilian Employees Drug Abuse Testing Program.

Drug-free federal workplace: Executive Order 12564. (1986, September 15). *Federal Register.*

Drug-Free Workplace Act of 1988, P.L. 100-690, Subtitle D. (1988, November).

Drug testing gains support. (1989, May 24). *The Sacramento Bee.*

Drug testing increasingly becoming standard procedure at workplace, (1984, August 5). *Baltimore Sun.*

Drugs in the Workplace: Research and Evaluation Data. (1989). (NIDA Research Monograph 91). Washington, DC: U.S. Department of Health and Human Services.

Drugs on the job. *Time,* (1986, March 17), p. 52.

Drug tests for all? (Editorial). (1986, March 14). *The Washington Post,* p. A18.

Drug tests get harder union look. (1986, October 19). *Newsday Business.*

Epilepsy Foundation of America. (1986, May 18). Written statement of position on drug testing, Board of Directors.

Equal Employment Advisory Council: Update of state and local legislative proposals regarding drug testing. (1987, June 11). Memorandum (87-82) to EEAC members from Kenneth McGuiness, president.

Getting tough on drugs. (1983, December 5). *U.S. News & World Report,* p.85.

Hansen, H.J., Caudill, S.P., & Boone, J. (1985). Crisis in drug testing: Results of CDC blind study. *Journal of the American Medical Association, 253*(16), 6–11.

Hartness vs. *Bush.* (1989, May 19).

Harwood, H.J., Napolitano, D.M., Kristiansen, P.L., & Collins, J.J. (1984). Economic costs to society of alcohol and drug abuse and mental illness: 1980. Research Triangle Institute: Research Triangle Park, NC.

House Select Committee on Narcotics (1981). *Results: Personal drug use survey* (study mission to Italy and the Federal Republic of Germany), U.S. House of Representatives. Washington, DC: U.S. Government Printing Office.

Krauthammer, Charles, (1985, August 9). Drug abuse: The supply-side approach. *The Washington Post,* p. A23.

Krauthammer, Charles, (1986, April 11). Drug testing? Choose liberty instead. *The Washington Post,* p. A15.

Lancaster, J. (1987, January 23). Amtrak head calls for drug testing. *The Washington Post,* p. A5.

Marcus, R., & Engel, M. (1986, February 2). Many employers testing workers for drug use. *The Washington Post,* p. 1.

National Foundation for the Study of Employment Policy. (1989). Matrix of State and Local Drug Testing Requirements.

National Organization for the Reform of Marijuana Laws (NORML), FDA petition. (1986, September).

National Transportation Safety Board (1983).

NTEU vs. *von Raab,* Civil Action No. 86-3522, US District Court for Eastern Louisiana. (1986, November 11).

NTEU vs. *von Raab,* 816 F. 2d 170 (5th Cir. 1987), US Supreme Court.

O'Boyle, T.F. (1985, August 8). More firms require employee drug tests; legal questions surround spread of mandatory screening. *The Wall Street Journal,* p. 6.

President's Commission on Organized Crime. (1986, March). *America's Habit: Drug Abuse, Drug Trafficking, and Organized Crime,* Report to the President and Attorney General.

Public Law 100-71, sec. 503, title IV (1987, July 11). *Congressional Record,* (vol. 133).

Report on drugs in the workplace (1983, August 22). *Newsweek,* pp. 52–59.

RLEA vs. *Burnley,* 88-4824 CAL (9th Cir. 1988), US Supreme Court.

Stille, A. (1986, April 7). Drug testing: The scene is set for a dramatic legal collision between the rights of employers and workers. *The National Law Journal.*

Subcommittee on Civil Service of the House Committee on Post Office and Civil Service. (1986, June). Patricia Schroeder, chairwoman, staff study.

Testing for drugs; tested by drugs (Editorial). (1986, March). *The New York Times,* p. A20.

USA Today poll. (1986, March 7). *USA Today,* p. 7.

U.S. Court of Appeals: *Borsari* vs. *Federal Aviation Administration,* 1983.

U.S. Department of Health and Human Services. (1988, April 11). *Mandatory guidelines for federal workplace drug testing programs. Federal Register.*

U.S. Department of Labor. (1989, January 11). New survey measures extent of drug-testing programs in the workplace.

Yes: Drug tests for (some) officials. (1988, July 12). *The New York Times.*

3

Common Drugs of Abuse: Pharmacology and Phenomenology

RONALD M. PAOLINO

A rational approach to both drug testing in the workplace and treatment of identified abusers requires a basic knowledge of the pharmacological principles of drug action. It is also important for managers, supervisors, and treatment providers to have an understanding of the specific characteristics of commonly abused drugs, for signs and symptoms are often specific indicators of the drug used. The ability to recognize drug-induced symptoms and withdrawal effects is essential in identifying drug use in the workplace as well as providing effective treatment. To this end, the focus of this chapter is directed at managers and supervisors as well as those individuals who counsel drug abusers. It is not intended to be a technical exposition of the biochemical and physiological effects of drugs. Readers who are interested in more in-depth scientific explanations and studies on the topics discussed are directed to the list of sources at the end of the chapter.

Commonly abused drugs or classes of drugs are discussed. In addition to general data, information is also presented concerning route of administration; symptoms and effects; acute toxicity; whether or not withdrawal and tolerance are observed; and what to look for in suspected users.

BASIC PRINCIPLES OF PHARMACOLOGY APPLICABLE TO DRUG ABUSE

Drugs produce their action by either stimulating or depressing already existing bodily functions and are incapable of producing new effects. Proponents of the "drop out, tune in, and turn on" drug culture of the 1960s often made claims that hallucinogens, such as LSD and mescaline, were capable of generating creativity and insight. Many gullible individuals took these drugs hoping to be so transformed only to find that the perceived "insights" disappeared as the effects of the drug wore off.

The potency of the drugs abused varies widely, ranging from microgram quantities for LSD to gram amounts in tolerant benzodiazepine abusers. One therefore needs to assess the amount and frequency of drug used in comparison to "normal" doses (particularly in prescribed medications) rather than to compare amounts used between various classes of drugs.

Drugs can produce a number of effects. Pharmacological or desired effects are those primary effects for which the drug is prescribed and intended. Drugs are also capable of producing undesirable effects or side effects at normal dosages. Adverse effects can be either idiosyncratic or dose related—that is, increase in frequency as the dose of the drug is increased. Toxic or lethal effects result as the drug dosage is increased further. Abusers and addicts usually take drugs for what are normally considered to be side effects. For example, benzodiazepines, normally taken for their anti-anxiety properties, may actually be abused for their memory-impairing effect. This means that abusers invariably take amounts closer to the toxic end of the dosage range.

The first step in drug intake involves absorption. Before any drug can have a psychotropic effect, it must be absorbed into the bloodstream and transported to the brain. Once into the blood, the drug is subject to a number of processes, the first of which is possible binding to blood proteins. Generally speaking, for a psychotropic drug to be active it must be in the free or unbound state. As such, the unbound drug undergoes translocation, which may involve deposit into storage depots. The rapidity of uptake into storage is dependent primarily on the water/oil solubility of the drug. The more oil-soluble the drug, the more rapidly it is taken up into fat and muscle tissue, thereby decreasing the amount circulating in the blood and available to the brain. A primary example of this action involves ultra-short-acting barbiturates such as thiopental, which must be given intravenously. The duration of action is on the order of minutes because of the extremely rapid uptake of the drug into muscle and fat tissue.

Uptake into fat tissue may prolong drug action, since drugs stored in fat slowly redistribute into the blood, resulting in sustained low blood levels. The rate of redistribution is determined primarily by the oil/water solubility equilibration constant for the drug. Conditions altering this equilibration, such as blood pH or fat mobilization resulting from stress or diet, may cause a sudden increase in blood concentrations of fat-stored drugs. It has been hypothesized that sudden release of highly fat-soluble PCP may account for drug-related effects weeks or months after the drug is ingested.

Drugs circulating in the blood are also subject to biotransformation, the process of metabolism in the liver. While most drugs are metabolized to inactive forms, there are instances where apparently inactive compounds are transformed to active metabolites in the body. The overall physical-biochemical effect of metabolism is to increase the water solubility of drugs, thereby facilitating excretion in urine.

In summary, duration of drug action depends on a number of factors, including protein binding in blood, translocation, storage, biotransformation, and rate of excretion. The time required for the amount of drug in the body to be reduced by 50 percent is described as the biological half-life of the drug ($t_{1/2}$).

ROUTES OF ADMINISTRATION COMMONLY USED BY DRUG ABUSERS

The route of administration used by the drug abuser will determine how rapidly and how much of the drug will get into the bloodstream. For many drugs of abuse—for example, heroin and cocaine—the "rush" or initial intense physical and psychological feeling is directly related to getting as much of the drug into the bloodstream as quickly as possible. Oral administration results in slow and incomplete absorption. This route is usually used with prescribed medications or when the abuser is looking for a sustained action rather than a rush. Onset of action with intravenous (IV) administration is extremely rapid since the process of absorption is bypassed. "Booting," a common practice of IV drug users to intensify the rush, consists of drawing small amounts of blood into the syringe, mixing it with drug solution, and injecting the mixture into the bloodstream. The procedure is repeated over and over until the entire syringe full of drug is injected.

Inhalation of drugs in the form of smoke or vapor produces an extremely rapid absorption essentially equivalent to IV injection. This is not surprising when one considers that the alveolar surface area of one lung in contact with circulating blood is equivalent to the area of a tennis court. Absorption from intramuscular injection, although slower than IV, is also rapid. This route is usually used by IV abusers whose superficial veins have collapsed owing to repeated use. Absorption through direct contact of the drug with mucous membranes (i.e., sniffing) is also rapid. While commonly associated with cocaine use, many drugs are taken by this route. Epidermal injection, also known as "skin popping," is used where both a slow absorption and sustained release of the drug are desired.

COMBINATIONS OF DRUGS

Most drug abusers use more than one drug. When an individual is identified as using a given drug, it can be assumed with reasonable certainty that other substances are also being used. Polydrug abuse is the rule rather than the exception. Combinations of drugs are used for a variety of reasons. Abusers or addicts are "connoisseurs" of the psychotropic effects of drugs. Drugs are chosen for a specific action desired at a given time.

Drugs may be taken in combination in order to "boost" or augment a desired action. An example is the use of Valium with opiates. Augmentation is possible because of the pharmacological phenomena of *addition* and *potentiation*. In the first instance, the overall effect is the simple sum of the actions of the individual drugs taken. In the latter (potentiation), the combination of effects is greater than the sum of the effects of the individual drugs. Within a medical context, potentiation allows for the decrease in dose of a drug to produce a therapeutic effect. For example, Atarax is used to potentiate the analgesic action of Demerol in the control of pain. However, polydrug use in the abuser can, and frequently does, result in a lethal overdose. Drugs may be used in tandem or in combination in order to counteract unwanted effects. Cocaine addicts often use central nervous system depressants, such as opiates, to control hyperstimulation.

COMMON DRUGS OF ABUSE

Marijuana

General

Marijuana is second only to alcohol in popularity. It is estimated that two-thirds of young adults 18 to 25 years of age have used it and that one out of four individuals in this age range currently uses marijuana. The drug, which comes from the Indian hemp plant *Cannabis sativa,* is found in temperate areas throughout the world. While there are sixty related compounds found in the plant, the principal active ingredient is delta-9-tetra-hydrocannabinol (THC). The concentration of THC varies from 1 percent to 6 percent and may reach as high as 10 percent. The higher concentrations are found in the female plant. There are a variety of cannabis preparations: bhang (India); Acapulco Gold, Panama Red, and Black Ganja (Africa); "Maui Wowi" (Hawaii); and Sinsemilla among others. While abusers may refer to buying pure THC ("tea") on the street, in point of fact this compound is not available in that form. The most common substitute is phencyclidine (PCP). Medically, marijuana has been used in the treatment of asthma, glaucoma, and nausea associated with cancer chemotherapy.

How Taken

Dried marijuana leaves, seeds, and flowers are usually smoked in a pipe or cigarette. They may be ground up and mixed with food, such as cookies or brownies, or put into drinks.

Symptoms/Effects

In the early stages of intoxication, the user appears animated. Speech tends to be loud with a great deal of giddiness. This phase eventually gives

way to a more subdued state in which the individual may appear sleepy.
Users may experience a sense of unique insight and fascination in commonplace objects and occurrences, which disappears when the drug
wears off. Time perception is significantly slowed down and it is common
for a user to feel as if time is "standing still." There is often a distortion
in depth perception. Motor performance efficiency is decreased with
complex tasks being affected to a greater extent. These effects can last
up to twenty-four hours after smoking one marijuana cigarette. Users may
also experience distortion in both sight and sound.

While euphoria and uncontrollable laughter are the more common effects, marijuana users, particularly inexperienced and anxious ones, may
experience brief, mild paranoid reactions. Occasional acute and intense
panic reactions are reported by both experienced and inexperienced
users.

Physiological effects accompanying marijuana use include increased heart
rate, dry mouth, and reddening of the eyes. Increased hunger, referred to by
users as "the munchies," and increased thirst are also common.

Tolerance/Withdrawal

There is no clear evidence for either physical dependence or withdrawal
resulting from cessation of marijuana use. However, many regular users
appear to develop a psychological dependence on the drug in which smoking becomes an integral part of daily living. The author has treated a number of individuals who smoked 15 to 20 marijuana cigarettes a day. A clear
tolerance to the effects of the drug had been developed. These individuals
were able to stop without showing any signs of withdrawal. One person
resumed because not smoking had left a "void" in his daily monotonous
routine.

Acute Toxic Effects

There are no acute physiological toxic reactions to marijuana. The most
likely adverse psychological reaction is paranoid thinking or panic reaction. When this occurs it is best treated by a calm, supportive approach
until the person returns to a normal state.

What to Look for in Suspected Users

It is often difficult to identify the casual marijuana user by behavior, out-
ward physiological effects, or affect. Common signs are reddened eyes
and uncontrollable or inappropriate laughter. However, it should be noted
that users easily mask the ocular effects by using over-the-counter eye
drops.

Cocaine
General

Cocaine is the active alkaloid obtained from the plant *Erythroxylon coca*.
The primary source of the drug is South America, principally Colombia,

Peru, and Bolivia. An estimated 80 percent of all cocaine entering the United States comes from the Medellin cartel in Colombia. Until as recently as 1975 cocaine was ranked as a lesser drug problem, and "experts" considered the drug to be benign. However, by 1986 cocaine was described as the fastest-growing drug problem in the United States and a major epidemic. Cocaine has been ranked as comparable to the fifth largest business among Fortune 500 companies. It has been estimated that as many as 30 million Americans have tried cocaine and perhaps 2 million to 4 million are addicted to the drug. The number of people seeking treatment has steadily increased over the years. Cocaine is commonly used with alcohol, and for many individuals, drinking alcohol is the "trigger" that initiates cocaine use. When this is the case, it is crucial to eliminate the use of alcohol if the individual is to stop using cocaine.

An increase in the availability and purity of cocaine, along with decreased price, has made cocaine a major drug of abuse in this country. There is a great deal of violence associated with the cocaine trade. This is attributable to the extremely lucrative nature of the cocaine "business" coupled with the pharmacological action of the drug, which increases aggressive behavior.

How Taken

Cocaine enters the body through a number of routes. It can be sniffed. This is done by dividing a quantity of cocaine powder into "lines": ten to twelve lines are usually obtained per gram of powder. Absorption from the nasal mucous membrane is incomplete (50 to 60 percent), with the onset of action being 3 to 5 minutes. Cocaine can also be injected intravenously, with the onset of the "high" occurring within seconds. The drug can be smoked in the forms of "free-base" or "crack," which are created by converting the cocaine hydrochloride salt to cocaine, the free alkaloid base. Free-base and crack differ only in the method of preparation. The term *crack* is derived from the crackling sound that is made when the substance is heated, probably due to the baking soda used in its preparation. While cocaine hydrochloride vaporizes at 195°C, free-base or crack does so at 98°C, making inhalation possible. Absorption is rapid, similar to IV injection, and essentially 100 percent. Subjective effects are experienced within seconds. However, the intense euphoria is short-lived, causing the user to smoke more in an attempt to regain the original high. Because this does not happen, the user continues to "chase the dragon" by increasing the frequency and quantity of free-base or crack use.

Symptoms/Effects

The high from cocaine consists of a euphoria of such intensity that addicts are often at a loss for words to describe it to nonusers. Some have described it as a "total body orgasm" lasting several minutes accompanied by a feeling of well-being, self-confidence, and invulnerability. When the drug wears off the user feels "let down" and depressed.

Regular cocaine use is accompanied by restlessness and hyperactivity. The user may be extremely talkative with an intense speech pattern. Mood swings are common, alternating between depression and euphoria. Sniffling and nasal congestion are seen in the occasional user. Ulceration of the nasal septum is often present in the chronic user. Weight loss is produced by the appetite suppressant action of the drug. A general irritability is seen in which the individual becomes annoyed or angry at the slightest provocation. Occasionally, one may observe blemishes on the face or arms that are the result of picking at the skin, owing to the feeling of "bugs" crawling under the skin.

Physiologically, cocaine produces dilated pupils and increased body temperature. Effects on the cardiovascular system include constriction of peripheral blood vessels with an increase in both blood pressure and heart rate. A significant number of deaths have been reported from cardiac arrest.

Heavy use is accompanied by paranoid thinking, with delusions that others are planning to attack or kill the user. Hallucinations may also be present. It is not uncommon to hear reports of heavy users locking themselves inside their homes, drawing the curtains, and hiding behind furniture with a loaded firearm waiting for some imagined aggressor to come after them. The chances of violence are extremely high in such instances. As the drug wears off, an intense feeling of self-disgust may result in such individuals turning the weapon on themselves. Bouts of intense, continual use ("runs") are often followed by feelings of self-contempt and low self-esteem accompanied by an overwhelming sense of guilt. Heavy use is invariably accompanied by severe financial problems because of the cost of the drug. Acquiring funds is accomplished in many ways. Dealing cocaine to others is common though usually not sufficient. Many middle-class and upper-middle-class users resort to "white collar crime" such as embezzling, while poorer users get involved in activities such as robbery and car theft. The existence of credit cards has led many abusers to use this mode of exchange as a way of obtaining cash for their drugs.

Tolerance/Withdrawal

As previously mentioned, cocaine was initially thought to be nonaddictive. It is currently estimated that perhaps 10 percent of all casual users go on to develop a serious cocaine habit. However, there is no way to predict who such individuals are.

The initial underestimation of the pernicious nature of cocaine use was exacerbated by the definition of addiction derived from opiate drugs, which emphasized the phenomena of tolerance, physical dependence, and withdrawal—phenomena not readily seen with cocaine. The lack of clear signs of withdrawal caused many people to conclude that cocaine was not addictive. However, with the current greater emphasis on the compulsive behavior and functional aspects (adverse consequences) associated with continued use, it has become obvious that cocaine is indeed one of the most addictive of the drugs of abuse.

Abrupt cessation of the use of large amounts of cocaine, particularly free-base or crack, results in a number of symptoms, which begin 24 to 48 hours after cessation and last 7 to 10 days. These symptoms can include severe depression, headaches, irritability, sleep disturbances, inability to concentrate, lack of motivation, and gastrointestinal upset. An intense period of suicidal ideation may be experienced during this time. Within two weeks of stopping the drug, the addict may report feeling totally free of the need for cocaine and express sincere and heartfelt intentions never again to use the drug. Those experienced in treating cocaine addicts know, however, that at this time the abuser is particularly vulnerable to relapse. If the person is being treated as an inpatient and is given a leave pass during this time, ward staff should not be surprised if the individual returns having used cocaine.

Acute Toxic Effects

Potential acute toxic effects include psychosis, paranoia, violent behavior, myocardial infarctions, cerebral-vascular accidents (strokes), aortic dissection, and cardiac failure. Convulsions resistant to benzodiazepines are also seen. Respiratory depression following convulsions is intensified by heroin, which is often used in combination with cocaine ("speedball").

What to Look for in Suspected Users

Cocaine users tend to exhibit psychomotor agitation and increased talkativeness. While on cocaine, the user's mood is characterized by elation, grandiosity, and increased irritability. Pupils are dilated and there may be nasal congestion. Extensive use is accompanied by suspiciousness or paranoia as well as an increased propensity toward violence.

Benzodiazepines
General

For the past twenty-five years benzodiazepines have been considered the drugs of choice for treating anxiety. Known as *anxiolytics,* these drugs have been the most commonly prescribed of the psychotropic medications. Of the top two hundred medications prescribed in 1986, Valium (diazepam) and Xanax (alprazolam) ranked eighth and twelfth, respectively. In 1988, Valium dropped in rank to twenty-seventh, and Halcion (triazolam), a new benzodiazepine, ranked sixteenth. Xanax was third after amoxicillin (an antibiotic) and Lanoxin (a cardiac medication). The widespread use of anti-anxiety drugs speaks to the nature of present-day society. While most of these drugs are remarkably safe even when taken in overdose quantities, clinicians working in the field of addiction will readily attest to their abuse liability. The problem of benzodiazepine dependency is exacerbated by the tendency for harried physicians, particularly general practitioners, to overprescribe these drugs, which is prompted by pressure from patients to get "something" for vague complaints of pain and emotional upset.

For general purposes of discussion, the benzodiazepines may be divided into short ($t_{1/2}$ = 4 to 20 hours) and long ($t_{1/2}$ = 24 to 72 hours) half-life compounds. Examples of short half-life compounds are lorazepam (Ativan), temazepam (Restoril), oxazepam (Serax), alprazolam (Xanax), and triazolam (Halcion). Examples of long half-life compounds are chlordiazepoxide (Librium), clorazepate (Tranxene), diazepam (Valium), flurazepam (Dalmane), and clonazepam (Clonopin).

How Taken

The benzodiazepines are taken orally either alone or in combination with other drugs. In the latter instance, they are used either to potentiate the euphoric action of drugs such as heroin or methadone, or to minimize unwanted side effects such as hyperexcitability produced by cocaine.

Symptoms/Effects

Benzodiazepines decrease anxiety and produce muscle relaxation. Sedation and transient memory impairment become pronounced as the dose is increased. Suppression of seizure activity is a common effect. Higher than normal doses result in slurred speech, ataxia, and impaired psychomotor performance. A decrease in aggressive behavior is usually seen, although the disinhibiting effects of diazepam may at times cause an actual increase in aggression in violence-prone individuals.

Tolerance/Withdrawal

A definite tolerance and physical dependence is seen in individuals who have abused high doses of benzodiazepines for long periods of time. The author has treated numerous individuals with diazepam habits of 500 to 600 mg a day. The average prescribed dose is 5 mg two or three times a day.

Abrupt cessation from high doses of benzodiazepines results in a withdrawal pattern similar to that seen with the barbiturates. Withdrawal from the shorter half-life compounds develops more dramatically and acutely, generally emerging within two days and terminating within a week. Withdrawal from longer half-life agents begins within two to three days, peaking within four to five days, and ending two to four weeks after onset. Rebound insomnia and anxiety are more likely to be noted with the shorter half-life drugs. The withdrawal syndrome includes agitation, insomnia, tremulousness, gastrointestinal upset, sweating, and nausea. There is also an increased sensitivity to light and sound. Benzodiazepine detoxification should be conducted on an inpatient basis because of the possibility of major convulsions. This is particularly true if the individual has had a history of prior seizures. Detoxification consists of starting the patient at the pretreatment dose level and decreasing the amount given by 10 percent each day. Vital signs are carefully monitored.

Acute Toxic Effects

Benzodiazepine poisoning is rarely associated with severe cardiovascular or respiratory depression. Treatment consists of gastric lavage and general supportive measures.

What to Look for in Suspected Users

Individuals using high doses of benzodiazepines such as diazepam tend to present themselves in an argumentative manner. Speech is slowed or slurred, and lack of coordination or ataxia may be present. Individuals often forget what they are arguing about. Sedation or drowsiness is evident. Oftentimes, the person's face will have a "relaxed" appearance due to a decrease in facial muscle tone.

Opioids

General

For purposes of convenience this section will focus on heroin and its metabolite, morphine, since much of what is stated applies also to other natural, semisynthetic opioids—for example, codeine, hydromorphone (Dilaudid), and oxycodone (Percodan)—and synthetic opioids (e.g., meperidine (Demerol) and methadone). It is important to note that many individuals become iatrogenically (induced by treatment) addicted to narcotics prescribed for pain management on an outpatient basis. This is likely to occur when the prescribing of narcotics continues after the painful condition disappears.

Prolonged prescribing is encouraged by patients who pressure physicians with vague undiagnosable complaints of pain, requesting the continuation of medication. Many of these patients have adapted to a new drug-induced state of everyday existence which they consider "normal." The most difficult patients to treat are those who are both iatrogenically addicted and continue to be in sufficient chronic pain to require prescribed narcotics. The tendency to continue taking increased amounts of analgesic is compounded by the development of tolerance. It is interesting to note that individuals in significant pain who are administered narcotic analgesics in a controlled inpatient environment seldom become addicted. If anything, physicians and nurses tend to be overly conservative with narcotics for inpatients, which sometimes leads to these patients suffering needless pain.

While the street addict usually has a specific drug of choice, narcotics are substituted for each other when the drug of choice is not available. For example, a heroin addict may use Dilaudid or Percodan. Often the choice is determined by availability and cost.

How Taken

Opiates and related drugs can be taken intravenously (heroin, Dilaudid, Demerol), orally (Percodan, Vicodan, methadone, Dilaudid), can be smoked (opium), and taken intramuscularly. This latter route is often used by heroin addicts when all superficial veins have been exhausted.

Symptoms/Effects

The symptoms and effects seen with morphine are discussed because morphine may be viewed as a prototype for this class of drugs. In doses of 5 to 10 mg, voluntary movements are decreased and accompanied by a drowsiness from which the individual can be readily aroused. Euphoria is experienced along with a decrease in self-control. Pain perception is decreased and there may be occasional vomiting.

As the dose is increased (15 to 30 mg) one sees all of the above symptoms along with an increase in the depth of analgesia. Pupils are very constricted and appear pinpointed. Doses above 30 mg produce a coma-like state with decreased respiration, which, if untreated, will result in death. Respiratory depression is produced at all dose levels. While sedation and drowsiness are commonly seen, there are individuals who respond to morphine with behavioral excitation.

In the addict, morphine or heroin produces a general feeling of well-being and satiation in which hunger and sexual drives are diminished, accompanied by a feeling of relaxation and imperturbability. The initial "rush" from IV injection described by new addicts tends to be missing or minimal in the veteran addict. This latter group tends to indicate that the primary reason for using opiates is to avoid the pain and anguish of withdrawal, as well as to obtain a relaxed feeling.

Here it is also important to point out a phenomenon familiar to clinicians treating opiate addicts—namely, that of the addict who states he or she needs the opiate or methadone simply to feel "normal." Careful interviewing and experience treating these patients reveal that with a small group of addicts there appears to be no need to take these drugs other than to function normally in everyday life. When placed on regulated doses of methadone these individuals function well. One can speculate on the possibility of such individuals having a deficiency in endogenous opioidlike compounds for which they self-medicate with opiates.

Tolerance/Withdrawal

A clear and definite tolerance develops with continued use of the opiates. Within a hospital setting, tolerance to the analgesic and euphoric effects of morphine develops within one to two weeks of repeated subcutaneous injections of 10 to 15 mg doses given twice per day. Tolerance will last one to two weeks after the drug has been stopped. Tolerance does not develop, however, to the miotic effects or constriction of smooth muscle of the gastrointestinal and biliary tracts. The lack of tolerance development makes pinpoint pupils a good indicator for the presence of morphine. The increased intestinal muscle tone accompanied by decreased motility is the source of constipation seen in opiate abusers. Constriction of the bile duct may result in increased pressure pain as the analgesic effect of morphine wears off.

Physical signs of withdrawal become evident in the addict within eight to sixteen hours after the last dose. Symptoms include yawning, watery eyes and nose, and alternate hot and cold flashes. As withdrawal intensifies, additional signs are seen, including gooseflesh (particularly in the pectoral area), dilated pupils, loss of appetite, restlessness, irritability, and tremor. Blood pressure and pulse rate are elevated. These signs are accompanied by subjective complaints of deep muscle pain (particularly in the legs), anxiety, and insomnia. Withdrawal from heroin (morphine) reaches its peak within two to three days. During this time, one sees an exaggeration of all of the above symptoms accompanied by nausea, vomiting, abdominal cramps, and diarrhea. Symptoms decline within one week.

Observation of initial stages of withdrawal is one important criterion to verify a suspected opiate addict. This information, along with urinalysis results indicating the presence of opiates and fresh needle tracks (for IV users), provides sufficient objective data to conclude that the person is physically dependent upon opiates. In the event that it is not feasible to wait for withdrawal symptoms to develop, one may document physical dependence by precipitating withdrawal with the use of naloxone (Narcan), an opiate antagonist. Intramuscular administration of this drug will induce withdrawal in the opiate addict within minutes. Once observed, the withdrawal syndrome may be terminated with the administration of morphine.

Acute Toxic Effects

Acute opiate poisoning is accompanied by coma and severe respiratory depression in which the person may become cyanotic. Pupils are very constricted and do not react to light. Treatment includes ensuring that the patient has a clear airway and proper ventilation. A dramatic reversal may be obtained by the administration of naloxone. It is common to see a comatose opiate overdose patient suddenly sit up wide awake even before an injection of naloxone is completed. However, because of the much shorter duration of action of naloxone in comparison to the opiates, the patient must be carefully monitored to see that he or she does not lapse back into coma and die.

What to Look for in Suspected Users

Constricted or pinpoint pupils that respond slowly or do not react to light are a key sign of opiate abuse (the exception is Demerol, which produces dilatation). Shallow or depressed breathing may also be observed. One should look for fresh needle tracks, usually on the forearms. However, IV drug users are very creative in where they inject themselves so as to avoid detection. Veins in the legs, ankles, toes, or even the penis may be used. Veins hidden in the eyebrows are also a source. A characteristic dozing off, referred to as "on the nod," may be seen in individuals under the influence of opiates. In this state the user will fluctuate between wakefulness and dozing even in the middle of a conversation. The person may be readily aroused and appear alert only to begin dozing again within seconds.

Phencyclidine
General

Phencyclidine (PCP) was synthesized in the 1950s and marketed in the 1960s as an anesthetic for humans. Its use was discontinued in 1965 following reports of induced hallucinations, seizures, and delirium. The drug is presently used in veterinary medicine as an animal anesthetic. Discouraging the illicit production of PCP is difficult, for it is easily and inexpensively synthesized by amateur chemists and brings in enormous profits. On the street, the drug is commonly referred to as "angel dust."

PCP is often used as a substitute for tetrahydrocannabinol (THC) or as an additive to enhance the effects of other drugs (marijuana, cocaine). It is an extremely dangerous substance. While often referred to as a hallucinogen, its effects are more accurately described as schizophrenogenic because the observed effects are similar to those of schizophrenia. PCP users brought into the emergency room must be treated with extreme caution even if in an apparent coma, for they may suddenly bolt up from a stuporous state and become violent. Outbursts of violence can be triggered by environmental stimuli such as the sight of a police officer's uniform. There have been reports of sudden and unprovoked outbursts of violence in PCP users weeks or months after using the drug. This long-lasting effect may result from the sudden release into the bloodstream of PCP that has been stored in fat tissue.

How Taken

PCP can be sniffed, injected intravenously, taken orally, or smoked with marijuana.

Symptoms/Effects

As mentioned previously, many of the effects of PCP closely resemble schizophrenia. The user experiences a distortion of body image, sometimes feeling as if parts of the body are floating off into space. Hallucinations, both visual and auditory, may be experienced, often with the theme of Satan. The external world becomes a strange and frightening place (depersonalization). Time perception is distorted and sensitivity to external stimulation increased. Paranoid thinking can lead to striking out in self-defense.

Behavioral and physiological effects are characterized by analgesia, motor incoordination, and autonomic nervous system activation consisting of salivation, elevated blood pressure, and sweating. These latter effects are dose dependent. At a dose of 5 mg or less, there is a general agitation and difficulty with speech. Horizontal or vertical nystagmus (involuntary, spasmodic movements of the eyeball) is present along with the tendency to stare into space. At doses of 10 mg or greater, the person is likely to be comatose.

Tolerance/Withdrawal

There is neither physical dependence nor withdrawal symptoms associated with the use of PCP.

Acute Toxic Effects

The patient will be comatose and will likely be in hypertensive crisis. Respiratory arrest is common along with deep analgesia. There is no specific antagonist for PCP as in the case of opiates. Standard life support measures should be employed. Once awake and stable, the patient should be kept in a quiet, dark room to minimize stimulation. Unlike schizophrenia, symptoms related to PCP disappear within several days without the use of antipsychotic drugs. This characteristic may be used to make a differential diagnosis between the two conditions, since many PCP users presenting on an outpatient basis appear schizophrenic.

What to Look for in Suspected Users

Vertical or horizontal nystagmus and elevated blood pressure are key differential diagnostic symptoms of PCP use. These are usually accompanied by confusion and chaotic thought disturbances. The individual appears agitated, pale, and sweating. Speech is often impaired.

Barbiturates

General

This class of central nervous system depressants is derived from the same basic chemical structure (barbituric acid) and has four basic uses: sedatives, hypnotics (to induce sleep), anesthetics, and antiepileptics. The barbiturates are qualitatively similar in action, differing in dose, onset, and duration. The one exception is that not all barbiturates possess antiepileptic activity. Barbiturates are classified according to duration of action, ranging from ultra-short-acting, with a duration of minutes, for example, thiopental, to long-acting, with a duration greater than six hours, for example, barbital. Short-acting agents with durations of action up to three hours tend to be the most widely abused, for example, pentobarbital ("yellow jackets") and secobarbital ("red devils").

How Taken

Barbiturates are taken primarily by the oral route.

Symptoms/Effects

In normally prescribed doses, barbiturates produce sedation that may be accompanied by a decrease in mental acuity and by emotional lability. With increased dosage there is a noticeable slurring of speech along with ataxia (loss of muscle coordination in walking) and vertigo. Unintentional poisoning with barbiturates may occur because of the phenomenon of "automatism" resulting from confusion, impaired memory, and distortion of time perception.

Tolerance/Withdrawal

A marked tolerance and physical dependence develop with the continued use of barbiturates. Withdrawal from these agents can be life-threatening and should not be attempted on an outpatient basis. The time of onset for withdrawal symptoms varies according to the half-life of the drug. For example, in the case of amobarbital, an intermediate-acting agent (duration 3 to 6 hours), early symptoms of withdrawal may be seen 12 to 16 hours after the last dose at which time the individual begins to complain of agitation, restlessness, and increased anxiety. Fatigue later becomes evident along with nausea and vomiting. Withdrawal peaks between 2 to 3 days when grand mal seizures are likely, with possible death resulting. In contrast to the opiates, barbiturate withdrawal is difficult to reverse during the peak phase.

Proper detoxification of the barbiturate-dependent patient must begin with an accurate assessment of the average daily intake of the drug. The patient's self-report should not be used, since it may be inaccurate. Rather, the starting dose is determined by the "pentobarbital tolerance test." Detoxification is accomplished by decreasing the amount by 100 mg each day.

Acute Toxic Effects

Acute barbiturate poisoning is characterized by respiratory depression and a decrease in body temperature, blood pressure, and reflexes. The clinical syndrome resembles opiate overdose. However, unlike the opiates, there is no specific antagonist for the barbiturates, and administration of naloxone has no reversing effect. Treatment consists of gastric lavage, artificial respiration, and supportive treatment with close supervision. Hemodialysis may be necessary in the event of renal failure.

What to Look for in Suspected Users

The barbiturate abuser looks inebriated but does not smell of alcohol. The gait is ataxic and speech is slurred. Pupils are normal in size and react to light. Drowsiness is a common feature.

Hallucinogens

General

The most notable of these compounds is lysergic acid diethylamide (LSD), which was synthesized in 1938 from alkaloids obtained from cereal grain infected with ergot fungus. It was not until 1943 that the hallucinogenic activity of the drug was discovered accidentally. Initially described as producing symptoms similar to schizophrenia, LSD was used to produce a "model psychosis." However, it now appears that LSD effects are more analogous to symptoms of acute brain syndrome.

Mescaline and psilocybin are hallucinogens of plant origin. The first substance is derived from the peyote cactus (*Lophophora williamsii*) and is obtained from disclike buttons (mescal buttons) 20 to 50 mm in diameter that grow on the plant. Psilocybin is extracted from the *Psilocybe* mushroom. Historical records indicate that use of these drugs by Mexican Indians in religious ceremonies dates back to the sixteenth century.

Use of the above hallucinogens was popular among members of the counterculture during the 1960s and early 1970s. Other hallucinogenic substances, such as nutmeg and morning glory seeds, were discovered and used during this period of searching for chemically induced "enlightenment." In addition to naturally occurring drugs there are also synthesized agents such as DET (diethyltryptamine) and DMT (dimethyltryptamine), the latter also known as the "businessman's special" because of its brief duration of action. Recently, there appears to be an increase in the use of LSD.

How Taken

Hallucinogens are taken orally.

Symptoms/Effects

The effects of the above-mentioned hallucinogens are essentially similar to those of LSD, differing primarily in duration of action and dose. When taken in 50 to 100 μg quantities, LSD produces what may be described as a "short circuiting" of the senses. Sounds may be seen as colors. Visual hallucinations are characteristic. Rats and snakes may appear from nowhere, and people may suddenly appear and disappear in front of automobiles. Sensory illusions are also common; cars may seem to crumble like accordions only to pop back into shape. The moon can turn into a giant spider or a companion's face may suddenly melt like wax. Rapid changes in mood may be experienced with vascillations from fright to exhilaration. Perception of time and distance is distorted. A heightened sense of meaning and understanding occur with sudden "insight" into age-old riddles or with direct "contact" with God. There may be an intense wonderment about common things. Often there is an overwhelming sense of invulnerability and belief that the user has special powers such as the ability to fly or to stop cars. These distortions have resulted in numerous deaths.

Physiological responses are primarily autonomic in nature with dilated pupils, flushed face, sweating, chills, and trembling. Sensitivity to light and sound is also increased.

The pleasantness or unpleasantness of the LSD experience is greatly influenced by the user's state of mind and immediate surroundings. Mood prior to taking the drug, expectation of the effects, the user's companions, and familiarity with the environment all determine whether or not a "trip" is good. Bad "trips" are not uncommon, and flashbacks have been reported long after the drug has been taken.

Tolerance/Withdrawal

While there is no reported physical dependence to LSD, a strikingly rapid tolerance does develop. Threshold doses of 50 μg may increase to several thousand micrograms after several days of continued use. Cross-tolerance is noted to mescaline and psilocybin. Both tolerance and cross-tolerance rapidly disappear with discontinued use. There is no withdrawal syndrome associated with LSD.

Acute Toxic Effects

Toxicity to LSD is behavioral in nature—that is, bad trips. These are best treated by supportively being with the user and talking him or her "down." Medication is seldom necessary.

What to Look for in Suspected Users

As might be expected, bizarre behavior and confused thought processes are common. The individual's face may be flushed, and he or she will often complain of chills. Users often don dark glasses to avoid increased sensitivity to light and to hide dilated pupils.

REFERENCES

Clouet, D.H. (Ed.). (1986). *Phencyclidine: An update*. (National Institute on Drug Abuse Research Monograph 64). Rockville, MD: NIDA.

Clouet, D., Aschar, K., & Brown, R. (Eds.). (1988). *Mechanism of cocaine abuse and toxicity*. (National Institute on Drug Abuse Research Monograph 88). Rockville, MD: NIDA.

Gilman, A.D., Goodman, L.S., Rall, T.W., & Murad, F. (Eds.). (1985). *The pharmacological basis of therapeutics* (7th ed). New York: Macmillan.

Harris, L.S. (Ed.). (1988). *Problems of drug dependence, 1988*. (National Institute on Drug Abuse Research Monograph 90). Rockville, MD: NIDA.

Sharp, C.W. (Ed.). (1984). *Mechanisms of tolerance and dependence*. (National Institute on Drug Abuse Monograph 54). Rockville, MD: NIDA.

4

Techniques of Reliable Drug Testing

ROBERT E. WILLETTE

Most government agencies and many private employers have initiated drug-testing programs to assure work force reliability. Several programs have been in place for a number of years, although the vast majority have started since 1981. Because these programs impact on the livelihoods of individuals, it is important to understand how drug testing operates, or should operate, and how to select the appropriate drug-testing procedures and a competent testing laboratory.

This chapter was written for individuals with little background in drug-testing techniques. A more comprehensive presentation has been published by the National Institute on Drug Abuse (NIDA) (Hawks & Chiang, 1986).

TOOLS OF THE TRADE

Analytical Chemistry: The Basics

The primary task of the analytical chemist is to identify and, if required, to measure the amount of a specific chemical that may be present in a given sample. If the sample is taken from a biological specimen, such as blood or urine, the task can be quite formidable because of the presence of thousands of other substances in the sample.

To conduct such an analysis, the chemist must separate the chemical or drug of interest from all other chemicals present and characterize it in a manner that provides sufficient information to identify it with some degree of scientific certainty. In the area of drug testing of certain populations, like athletes or employees, this level of scientific certainty must meet the legal or forensic standard of "beyond a reasonable doubt." Testing in counseling situations is usually conducted at a somewhat lower standard.

Modern chemistry has provided the analytical chemist with two types of methods that allow the necessary separation and identification to be conducted in an efficient and cost-effective manner. These two major techniques are *immunoassays* and *chromatography*. To achieve a foren-sic-quality result, it has become required practice to use both of these techniques in combination. Other combinations may also be acceptable, but the typical drug-testing scenario employs an immunoassay as an ini-tial test (often called a "screen") followed by a chromatographic analysis.

Immunoassays: Advantages and Limitations

An immunoassay separates a specific chemical, or group of closely re-lated chemicals, away from everything else in the sample being tested, by attracting or binding that chemical to an antibody designed to recognize it. Using the same principle that is responsible for allergies and immuni-zations, chemists have learned how to produce antigenic material that contains specific drug molecules. When these are injected into an animal, the animal's immune system produces antibodies that "recognize" the drug that was attached to the antigen. The antibodies are then collected from the animal for use in the assay.

To complete the assay, some type of "marker" molecule must be added to indicate when a drug is present. This is accomplished by adding the drug attached to an enzyme or a radioactive or fluorescent molecule to the assay mixture. When the specific drug is present in the sample, it competes with the marker molecule for binding sites on the antibody, thus releasing the marker into the surrounding solution. The amount of marker displaced is proportional to the amount of drug present. This displace-ment can then be measured by an appropriate instrument, such as a spec-trophotometer or scintillation counter.

The most significant advantage of immunoassays is their sensitivity. This means that a properly formulated immunoassay can detect extremely small amounts of the specific drug of interest. In practice, this makes it possible to detect drug use for relatively long periods of time. The actual cutoff, or concentration above which the test response is said to be pos-itive, can be adjusted to almost any level desired. This enables one to establish different detection periods depending on program goals.

Another advantage of immunoassays is the ease at which they can be adapted to high volume and rapid testing. This greatly reduces the cost of screening for several drugs at the same time. While the older radioim-munoassays (RIA, the one that uses a radiolabeled marker) are fairly la-bor-intensive and not easily amenable to automation, newer immunoas-says, like EMIT (which uses an enzyme marker), can be fully automated with computer-driven panels and bar-code readers. This form of immu-noassay is also available in portable test kits that are widely used by the military and by many companies at remote locations.

It was stated above that immunoassays can be produced that are quite specific for a given drug or closely related group of drugs. This latter aspect imposes one of the limitations of immunoassays. For example, the antibodies used in immunoassays for amphetamines tend to bind to, or cross-react with, several drugs that share amphetamine's basic structure. This makes these assays "class" specific. Thus, a positive response from an amphetamine immunoassay generally indicates that one or more of the several amphetaminelike drugs is present. The confirmation test must then distinguish between these. Other immunoassays, such as that directed at the cocaine metabolite benzoylecgonine, are extremely specific and do not detect any other chemical, except for very high concentrations of cocaine itself.

The immunoassays for marijuana are directed at the major metabolite or breakdown product of delta-9-tetrahydrocannabinol (THC), which is the major psychoactive ingredient in marijuana and other cannabis products. The metabolite, THC-9-acid for short, is used to produce the antibodies for these assays and as the standard for calibrating the analysis. However, the antibodies, which are obtained from animals (such as rabbits or goats), tend to attract or "cross-react" to varying degrees with several other THC metabolites. Thus, a response in this assay measures the total of cross-reacting metabolites that are present. Nevertheless, this "total" response does reflect the relative amount of THC present in the system, with several limitations as described below.

Chromatography: Many Ways to Separate Drugs

The term "chromatography" has its origins in the Greek word *chromo* for color. The concept is related to the rainbow, which displays the colors that make up light by separating them. The process of chromatography, as used in analytical chemistry, takes advantage of the different properties of chemicals and drugs that permit them to be separated from one another. This can best be illustrated by describing the various separation steps that occur in the most highly regarded assay, gas chromatography/ mass spectrometry (GC/MS).

The GC/MS analysis starts with a rough separation through some type of extraction. This is a process in which the sample, for example, a portion of a urine specimen, is treated with certain specific chemicals that make the drug of interest less soluble in the urine. This form of the drug and other chemically similar molecules are then removed from the urine by shaking the urine with a solvent for which the drug is now more soluble. Or, as an ever-growing alternative, the treated urine sample can be passed through a solid that attracts the drug molecules. The drug can then be retrieved from the solvent or solid and concentrated to a very small residue. This extraction process serves a very important role in selectively removing the drug from the many other chemicals and water in the urine, thereby simplifying the next stage of the analysis.

The concentrated extract is dissolved in a small amount of solvent and injected, by means of a syringe, into the inlet of a long, narrow tube known as a *chromatographic column*. Sometimes the extract must be treated with other reagents to produce a so-called derivative that is more stable or volatile than the parent drug. The next separation that takes place is in the chromatographic column. Older columns were filled with a solid material, often coated with a high boiling liquid, that could attract or absorb the chemical components in the extract. Newer columns are coated on the inside with the liquid and contain no solid packing. These are usually extremely narrow and are called "capillary" columns.

The column is coiled up inside a heated oven and is so arranged that a stream of gas is allowed to flow through the column. When the extract is injected into the stream of gas, it is swept through the column. Each of the chemicals present in the extract will be attracted to the column packing to varying degrees. Therefore, some will pass through faster than others, which are held up by their attraction to the column. If the proper conditions are selected (this is all done by extensive experiments with known materials), the drug of interest will be separated away from all of the other components.

The next part of the assay is to somehow detect when each of the separated components emerges from the other end of the column. This can be done in several different ways. The best method makes use of a mass spectrometer (MS). As its name implies, this instrument can record on a meter a spectrum of the molecules entering it, separated according to their molecular weight or, to be more technically correct, their mass. Thus, as the desired drug molecules emerge from the column, the stream of gas containing them is directed into the MS, which separates all components present by their molecular weight. All chemicals have a specific molecular weight, which is not necessarily unique. That is, more than one chemical can have the same molecular weight, but each must have a unique structure. It is these differences in structure that permitted the different molecules to be separated in the extraction and the chromatography steps.

To further characterize the chemical or mixture of chemicals that emerges from the GC column, most mass spectrometers are operated in a mode that causes the molecules to break up or "fragment" into pieces. Under the same operating conditions, each unique chemical will give rise to the same fragmentation pattern, similar in concept to that of a chemical fingerprint. It is this additional fragmentation information that makes the MS detector so powerful. Because the fragmentation pattern can vary from instrument to instrument or from day to day, it is necessary always to run known standards along with any unknown samples in order to make the comparison.

Taken together, the extraction process, the chromatographic and mass separations, and the matching of fragmentation patterns all combine to provide unequivocal evidence that the drug or drug metabolite is present in the sample. One last requirement is that the concentration of the compound be measured. This is necessary in order to prove that the signals measured in the mass spectrometer are due to the drug and not to any "background noise" caused by the sample or the instrument. Thus, a cutoff is established based on experiments using samples containing known amounts of the drug. During actual analyses, known standards must be included in the analysis so as to establish the appropriate calibration to the magnitude of signals produced by the sample. To make this extremely accurate, an "internal standard" is added to the sample before it is extracted. This produces a fixed relationship between the drug and the internal standard. By comparing these ratios for the standards against that from a sample, the concentration can be calculated.

It should be noted that other chromatographic assays are in use and available for drug testing. The more common of these are thin-layer chromatography (TLC) and high-pressure liquid chromatography (HPLC). Because these two methods do not offer the same degree of accuracy as GC/MS or other MS methods, their use as confirmatory assays has been discouraged. It is important, however, to describe briefly their usefulness and applicability to employee drug-testing programs.

Thin-layer chromatography is one of the oldest of the chromatographic methods. Instead of carrying the extracted chemicals through a column of adsorbing material with a stream of hot gas, as in gas chromatography, the extract is separated by a solvent that is allowed to migrate up a plate or film that is coated with a thin layer of an absorbent. Similar principles apply to the process of separation, except that some chemicals, which cannot be readily volatilized, are more amenable to separation on a TLC plate than in the GC column, although there are certain limitations, as noted below.

As in gas chromatography, there must be some means of detecting the separated chemicals on the TLC plate. This is usually done by spraying the developed and dried plate with various reagents that cause the chemicals to appear as colored spots. With the correct choice of "spotting" reagents, many drugs can be identified by the colors they produce. This information, taken together with the distance the "spot" traveled along the plate, serves to provide sufficient information for identifying the drug or drugs that were present in the extract. As in the case of GC, known standards must be run alongside the unknown samples to serve as distance and color references.

There are major limitations to thin-layer chromatography. Experience has shown that TLC has less separating or discriminating power than GC, although it does provide color information in addition to the distance traveled. While this suggests that TLC results are considered presumptive or as corroborating, there are several TLC assays that have been so well studied that the results can be considered more conclusive. An example may be some of the high-performance TLC (HPTLC) assays for marijuana use, although even these are not universally accepted.

The combination of a positive immunoassay result and positive TLC result is widely used as sufficient evidence of drug use in many treatment and penal settings, since in most cases it takes multiple positive results and other evidence, such as possession of the drug, to cause penalties to be imposed. In an employment setting, especially where a single urine specimen may have adverse consequences, it is the consensus that the use of GC/MS is recommended or required. Some laboratories offer TLC as an intermediate confirmatory step, with the client electing to have the GC/MS analysis conducted if there is to be any adverse action taken. While TLC analyses are generally less expensive than GC/MS, the price difference is narrowing as the cost of mass spectrometers is dropping and their widespread use expanding.

Another widely recognized limitation to TLC is its generally lower sensitivity, that is, that it takes a larger amount of drug to be present to be detected on a TLC plate. This is especially troublesome with the more commonly used drugs of abuse, since they are taken in lower doses and, therefore, produce lower concentrations in the urine than other drugs. Nevertheless, TLC is still a popular and relatively inexpensive screening method for use on patients in drug-treatment programs, where the level of drug use is generally quite high and is more easily detectable. This is why immunoassay methods are favored for use in employment situations, where the level of drug use may be lower or less frequent, often escaping detection by the less sensitive TLC assays.

One application where thin-layer chromatography is still very useful is in the routine detection of the use of many psychoactive prescription drugs. Because immunoassays have not been developed for most of these drugs, coupled with the fact that they are taken in larger doses and produce high concentrations in the urine, TLC is a convenient method for detecting many of them, all at one time. Some employers, those who have employees in safety-sensitive jobs, such as transportation, chemical production, and gas and electric plants, have a legitimate concern about the use of such medications. Many of these employers require applicants and employees to report the use of such drugs even if they are under medical care. It is necessary to determine if the dosage is properly adjusted, and if the individual is stabilized on the drug and taking it according to the prescribing physician's instructions. In most instances, the detection of unreported use of such drugs will lead to some type of remedial action by the employer.

The last assay method to be mentioned is high-pressure liquid chromatography. HPLC is very similar to GC except that the extracted chemicals are carried through a special adsorbent column by a liquid or solvent under high pressure. This is particularly useful, or necessary in some cases, when very large or complex drugs, which cannot be volatilized or breakdown in the heated gas column, need to be analyzed. Two drugs that tend to fall in this category are LSD and the family of benzodiazepines (e.g., diazepam). HPLC is still widely used for confirming the identity of compounds producing positive results in immunoassays for benzodiazepines. This has been so because of the many drugs and overlapping metabolites found in urine specimens.

However, with recent advances in technology, there are GC/MS analyses now available for even these drugs. For example, the U.S. Navy has started to screen for LSD use and confirm these positive specimens with a GC/MS method. Another development is the coupling of a mass spectrometer detector to an HPLC to take advantage of the added sensitivity and accuracy of the MS.

REQUIREMENTS FOR A RELIABLE DRUG-TESTING SYSTEM

Specimen Collection

One of the most critical factors in a reliable drug-testing program is the first step—that is, collecting the specimen. Since this is usually a urine specimen, it is necessary to have available a suitable facility to conduct the collection. There is considerable controversy about whether or not the collection should be witnessed. The need for witnessing is based on the well-known "tricks" of drug users who are very adept at substituting a "clean" specimen or adding an adulterant, such as water or chemicals, that could interfere with the testing. On the other hand, a majority of employers, including the nonmilitary agencies of the federal government, have chosen to permit the individual to provide the specimen in private. However, to guard against the possibility of adulteration or substitution, certain precautions must be taken.

The actual collection site is usually separate from the testing laboratory, but it may be part of the laboratory, either at the same or a remote location, or it can be located at the employer's place of business. National health care and paramedical service organizations offer collection services, either at their locations or at sites designated by the client.

The collection site must possess all necessary personnel, materials, equipment, facilities, and supervision to provide collection, security, storage, and transportation (shipping) of urine specimens to the contract laboratory. It must have bathroom facilities (commode, urinal, washstand with only cold water, soap, and paper towels) which are clean, well lit, and sufficiently secure to prevent compromise during the collection of urine specimens.

The collection site facility shall be secure at all times. Chain-of-custody forms must be properly executed by authorized personnel upon receipt of specimens. The handling and transportation of urine specimens from one authorized individual, or place, to another must always be accomplished through the use of chain-of-custody format. No unauthorized personnel shall be permitted in any part of the area where urine specimens are collected or stored.

All employees must wash and dry their hands thoroughly prior to urination in order to remove possible chemicals sequestered under the fingernails. Specimens shall be collected under the supervision of authorized personnel in temporary "catch" containers. Employees providing urine specimens shall not let the containers out of their sight until the specimen is transferred and sealed into the shipping bottle, as described below, by collection site personnel. It may be possible to collect specimens directly in the shipping bottle.

Immediately after collection, authorized personnel shall conduct a close inspection of each specimen in order to determine the specimen's warmth, color, and signs of contaminants. Any unusual findings resulting from the inspection must be included on the chain-of-custody form. Under certain circumstances, the collection site personnel may be required to measure the temperature of the specimen. Irrespective of the suspicious nature of the specimen, the specimen should still be forwarded for testing, since it may still test positive. Nevertheless, a second specimen should then be obtained under direct observation.

Following inspection, the specimen will be immediately poured into a "specimen" container, which must be shatterproof. The container will then have the cap tightly affixed and the cap sealed with approved "security tape" or "sealable bag." The employee must then initial the tape or sealed bag.

If the employee is unable to provide a specimen at the time of arrival at the collection site, he or she shall be given the opportunity to remain in the area of the collection site until the necessary specimen is provided. If an employee fails, for any reason, to provide the necessary specimen, or if the employee fails to appear at the site at the assigned time, such failure shall be noted on the chain-of-custody form.

Chain of Custody

Before, during (unless the specimen is provided directly into the bottle), and after urination, collection site personnel shall always have the urine specimen container within sight. The containers shall be tightly capped and properly sealed and labeled. The labeling should include as a minimum: (1) the employee's Social Security or employee number, (2) the company or agency's name or code number, (3) the employee's initials, and (4) the time and date of collection. The site should maintain a logbook containing this information and the signatures of the employee and collection person. The logbook will facilitate the identification of the specimen provider.

An approved chain-of-custody form shall be utilized as a method of tracking for the purpose of maintaining absolute control and accountability from initial collection to final disposition of all specimens, and these forms shall always accompany the specimens. The form will identify the specimens through use of information that matches label items as previously described and a sequential number, which is assigned by the laboratory to each urine specimen in each batch. With each transfer of possession, the chain-of-custody form must be signed and dated (including the time) by authorized individuals charged with possession of the specimens. Every effort must be made to minimize the number of people handling the specimens in order to simplify and tighten the overall security of the specimens.

After the site has collected, sealed, and labeled the specimens, collection site personnel shall arrange for reliable transportation (shipment) to an approved laboratory. If specimens are not to be shipped immediately, they must be stored in a locked, limited-access area. If they have to be housed overnight, they should be placed in a refrigerator. If the site proposes to utilize an in-house courier or other similar means to transport specimens, such service must be approved by the company or agency. When the approved service picks up urine specimens from the collection site for delivery to the laboratory, the chain-of-custody forms or other transfer forms (some laboratories require that the original chain-of-custody form be sealed in the bag with the specimen) must be signed by delivery personnel and receiving/accession personnel at the laboratory. The essential purpose of all of these signatures is to be able to establish who handled the specimen(s) at all times. Accusations of tampering are common and can be avoided with a comprehensive chain-of-custody system.

Reliable Laboratory

Another obvious requirement for a reliable drug-testing program is to use a laboratory that meets the highest standards of operation. Several factors determine the overall reliability of a laboratory. Some of the major ones will be described here. As shall be noted, there are laboratory accreditation and certification programs specifically designed for laboratories performing urine drug testing for employment purposes. It would certainly be prudent, and perhaps required, to use only such laboratories.

It is essential that the laboratory have a written manual outlining "standard operating procedures." The manual should include a detailed description of every step for specimen handling and analytical methods. Each page should be dated and signed to show that it is continually updated as the laboratory modifies procedures. It must explain everything the laboratory is doing to ensure that test results are properly reviewed and recorded.

In addition to the chain-of-custody procedures described earlier for the collection of specimens, the laboratory must very carefully maintain the chain of custody of specimens and test samples during the entire testing process. Employers should examine the documentation on chain-of-custody procedures from the time the specimens are collected until results are reported. Special handling procedures should be in effect for employee drug-testing specimens. These specimens should be separated from routine clinical specimens before sealed containers are opened.

After a container has been inspected it should be assigned a special identifying number, or accession number. This is the method for tracking the bottle, the request form, and the test result. Some laboratories place several copies of the same preprinted number on the specimen bottle.

These extra labels are used to identify test tubes containing the specimen or any other container. Bar-coded labels are now in use to ensure that accession numbers are not misread or entered incorrectly.

Integrity of the specimen is maintained by labeling specimen and aliquot containers, as mentioned previously. To maintain chain of custody, the original specimen container should never leave the secured or limited access part of the laboratory.

A completely new aliquot must be obtained from the original container when doing a confirmatory or any repeat test. Matching the numbers is essential in order to avoid mixing up the specimens. Only one specimen container can be open at any given time.

Who has access to stored specimens and why? How are they stored? Positive specimens should be stored frozen in a secure place and there should be a way to identify everyone who has had access to them. The laboratory should also be able to track exactly where each specimen was from the time it entered the laboratory until it was stored.

How are records and actual testing data stored? Who has access to them? They should be filed in an easily retrievable manner. The laboratory will have to provide notarized copies of all documents and data in any legal proceeding.

An agreement needs to be made with a laboratory about testing a specimen if there has been a flaw or an error in the handling of the specimen. In most cases, it is best to obtain a new specimen which cannot be faulted at a later date.

Laboratory staff must, at the very least, meet state requirements. These vary from state to state. The laboratory should have an internal certification program for each staff position and be certified or licensed by the state and one of the appropriate boards or societies.

The laboratory should be able to provide access to a well-informed staff capable of offering sound advice about drug testing, selection of appropriate cutoff levels, and interpretation of results.

In the event of legal or labor action, the laboratory must be able to defend a drug test in a hearing or in court through expert testimony. An expert witness who can defend testing methods and the scientific validity of results usually has a doctorate degree or considerable experience in the field of drug testing.

An important consideration in laboratory selection pertains to the materials the lab will supply. Most will provide all the specimen containers, request forms, evidence tape or sealers for the bottles, packaging materials (like plastic bags and boxes), and mailing or freight forms required for specimen collection. Some laboratories also include overnight courier delivery as part of their overall service.

Quality Assurance

It is a primary requirement for any laboratory to have in operation a quality assurance (QA) program. This should be comprehensive in that it provides constant surveillance of all aspects of laboratory operations, such as staff training and certification, preparation of reagents, internal chain-of-custody procedures, quality control, equipment functions and maintenance, and the reporting of results.

Quality control (QC) is a significant part of the QA program and is intended to ensure the accuracy of results by including samples with known concentrations with every batch of specimens that is analyzed. These samples are "open," or known to the operators, allowing them to evaluate the performance of each batch. Some laboratories include as many as 20 percent of each batch as QC samples. This number will vary with the test, the variability of the assay or equipment, and other factors. In addition, it is strongly recommended that the laboratory include blind samples among its quality control program.

The laboratory should make all of its QC data available for inspection along with evidence of its performance when it submits quality control samples through the laboratory on a "blind" basis. These blind samples can be obtained from another laboratory or a proficiency testing or quality control service. Review the quality control records. How are these samples introduced? Are blind samples truly indistinguishable to the technicians from regular specimens?

Reporting and Reviewing Results

It is important to understand and contract for specific turnaround times in the laboratory. Consider including a penalty clause, such as a 20 percent discount, for every day the results are delayed. Many laboratories provide results within 48 to 72 hours after specimen pickup. If confidential hard copies are needed immediately, some laboratories will set up an electronic means of transmitting results, other than the telephone. Telephoned reports should be avoided, for this method is least secure and most prone to mistakes. If urgency is not a factor, a mailed envelope, clearly marked "confidential," addressed to the person authorized to receive the results is adequate.

SELECTING A RELIABLE
DRUG-TESTING LABORATORY

Step One: Defining Your Needs

A number of important considerations should be reviewed when selecting a system for drug testing. The first major consideration is to decide whether testing will be done at the place of business ("on site") or by an outside laboratory. There are advantages to both systems. The second, and more important, consideration is the choice of laboratory used for confirmatory testing and/or all drug testing. Because services and prices vary significantly across laboratories, it is prudent to solicit proposals from several laboratories of known quality. Testing requirements should be spelled out to determine who is best able to provide them under the best terms. It is money well spent to pay a little more for better quality than to save a few dollars and have quality compromised. Challenged results and legal proceedings are far more expensive.

The only reliable method of testing depends on a confirmatory test of a positive result using an alternative method of testing. This should always be done by an outside laboratory if the screening is conducted in-house.

When setting out drug-testing requirements, several issues must be considered. Which drugs will be included? Most laboratories have various "panels" of drugs, each designed to meet different needs. For example, most employers select a drugs-of-abuse panel that includes marijuana, cocaine, amphetamines, opiates (heroin, morphine, codeine), PCP, and barbiturates. Many other employers add methaqualone, methadone, propoxyphene and benzodiazepines, if the abuse of these drugs is prevalent in their area. Immunoassays are available for all of these, as are GC/MS confirmation assays. They are usually available at a reasonable package price that includes all expenses. Most laboratories also offer comprehensive TLC, and a few laboratories GC and GC/MS, screens that complement the immunoassay panel. These assays can detect a whole host of other drugs that may be of concern (see above).

Another matter to decide is the cutoff point that determines when a positive result is to be reported as positive. Recall that each assay must have its minimum level of reliability established. This is the lowest concentration at which a sample would be reported positive. However, some arbitrary concentration above the minimum level can be set as the reporting cutoff point. This is done for a variety of reasons. For example, in the early days of the military drug-testing program, as many as 48 percent of enlisted personnel in the Navy admitted using marijuana on a regular basis, a figure verified by random urine tests at the 20 ng/mL cutoff. Had the Navy chosen the 20 ng/mL cutoff for routine testing, it would have detected more users than it could handle. Rather, the Navy (under Department of Defense authorization) chose to use a 100 ng/mL cutoff, which would detect more recent use, but obviously fewer individuals. The Navy compensated for this by subjecting everyone to frequent random testing. Thus, it encouraged most of the users to stop rather than be caught. The philosophy was: "Get rid of the abuse, not the abuser."

On the other hand, some employers—for example, those with workers in sensitive positions—have chosen to test less frequently but to use lower cutoffs. This helps to minimize the "false-negative" result, something that will occur more frequently with higher cutoffs. A false-negative result states that the sample is "negative" when the drug is actually present but below the cutoff point (or if it is above the cutoff point but the laboratory missed it for some reason).

There had been a tendency early in the period of drug testing of em-

TABLE 4.1 Common Assay Cutoffs

Drug Class	Cutoffs (ng/mL)
Initial test	
1. Marijuana metabolites	20, 50, 100
2. Cocaine metabolites	300
3. Opiates (morphine/codeine)	300
4. Phencyclidine (PCP)	25, 75
5. Amphetamines	300, 1000
6. Barbiturates	200
7. Methaqualone	300, 750
8. Benzodiazepines	300
GC/MS confirmation	
1. Marijuana metabolite[a]	10, 15
2. Cocaine metabolite(s)[b]	150
3. Morphine and/or codeine	300
4. Phencyclidine (PCP)	25
5. Amphetamine and/or methamphetamine	300, 500
6. Barbiturates	200
7. Methaqualone	300
8. Benzodiazepines[c]	300

[a]Delta-9-tetrahydrocannabinol-9-carboxylic acid.
[b]Benzoylecgonine, ecgonine methyl ester, and/or ecgonine.
[c]Usually as oxazepam, a common metabolite for several drugs.

ployees to use higher cutoffs in order to minimize or eliminate the possibility of a "false positive," that is, reporting that a drug was present when it wasn't. With the common availability of GC/MS as a confirmation method, which has reduced the possibility of false-positive results, more and more employers and laboratories are going to lower cutoffs. Even the Navy is pursuing the use of a lower cutoff for marijuana, since it has reduced its level of drug use in the enlisted ranks from the 48 percent figure in 1981, or 38 percent in 1983 (when testing at the 100 ng/mL cutoff began), to a rate of detection of nearly 1 percent in 1990.

Table 4.1 lists the more common cutoffs used for the initial test (immunoassays) and GC/MS confirmation for common drugs of abuse.

Laboratory Certification and Accreditation Programs

There is an official registry of certified laboratories that is published in the *Federal Register*. The Department of Health and Human Services (HHS) directed the National Institute on Drug Abuse (NIDA) to develop standards for performance (proficiency) testing and certification of labo-

ratories engaged in drug testing for federal agencies and employers covered by drug-testing regulations issued by the Department of Transportation and the Nuclear Regulatory Commission (Bowen, 1988). Other
similar regulations are pending from the Department of Defense and the
Department of Energy. The certification program began in October 1987,
with 52 laboratories certified through July 1990. Even if a company is not
required by regulation to use one of these certified laboratories, it is
strongly advised to do so. Whether certified or not, it is essential to understand what to look for in selecting the best laboratory available. The
factors described above should help.

Find out from federal and state agencies if the laboratory has been licensed in any government programs and how the laboratory performed.
Only California, New York, and Pennsylvania have proficiency testing
programs for drug-testing laboratories, although these programs differ significantly. Many other states have implemented stricter standards for this
type of testing. Check with your state to see if there are any special reg-
istration or licensure requirements. You may also want to get recommendations from experts in the field of drug-testing programs.

Inspection

It is very important to inspect the laboratories that you are considering
to use for your drug testing. Observe the organization and procedures for
processing specimens. Look for all of the critical factors described here.
See the chapter Appendix for an abbreviated sample checklist that may
be useful.

MONITORING THE LABORATORY

Proficiency Testing

The laboratory should be participating in at least one, and preferably all,
of the proficiency testing (PT) programs that are available. Many laboratories subscribe to one of the open surveys—that is, where samples are
sent directly to the laboratory—offered by the College of American Pathologists (CAP), American Association of Bioanalysts, or American Association for Clinical Chemistry (AACC). Both CAP and AACC offer a
combined program designed to accredit forensic-quality drug-testing laboratories; however, this program had not met federal standards by July
1990. Ask the laboratory if it participates in any of these and review the
results.

As noted earlier, the U.S. Department of Health and Human Services
provides PT monitoring of laboratories through a contract from NIDA as
part of its National Laboratory Certification Program. This involves the
shipment of 10 PT samples to certified laboratories every other month.

The spiking concentrations are targeted just above the minimum detection levels to assure a low rate of false negatives. Many negative samples are also included to check for false positives. Laboratories must maintain a 90 percent score on correctly identifying positives, no false positives, and quantitative results within 20 percent of reference laboratory values. This is considered a very rigorous program. Even if there is no legal requirement for using federally certified laboratories, it might be advisable to do so, as courts will generally want to know why you aren't using such a facility.

Blind Quality Control

Duo Research Inc. provides a blind quality control service to assist further in monitoring laboratory performance. In this program, the samples are sent to the client, who in turn submits them blind to the laboratory. This is a more rigorous method of determining how a laboratory does on a day-to-day basis when it does not know it is being tested. This service is supplemented with periodic laboratory inspections and reports.

INTERPRETATION OF RESULTS

What Does a Positive or Negative Result Mean?

Several factors determine whether or not a specimen will be reported positive for a drug. As previously noted, the choice of the detection cutoff or reporting level will clearly affect the meaning of the result. Generally, higher cutoff concentrations will detect more recent use and permit more drug use to go undetected. Other factors must also be considered in designing the drug-testing protocol and in reviewing and interpreting the results.

For example, the choice of specimen affects both the detectability of drug use and the interpretation. Blood tests are generally considered to provide more relevant information about recent use and possible impairment. This is because the concentration of drug circulating in the blood can be correlated with certain measures of impairment, at least for some drugs. But even here, no general consensus exists as to the degree of impairment and its relationship to a particular individual or job. Another problem with blood tests is that drug concentrations in blood are continually falling, usually rapidly, making the detection of most drugs very difficult. Furthermore, blood is a more difficult specimen to analyze; this makes analysis much more expensive than urine tests in many instances.

Because of the problems associated with blood tests, not withstanding the invasiveness of obtaining the specimen, urine is the preferred specimen for determining drug use. Drugs and/or their metabolites are excreted into urine, where they tend to accumulate and concentrate, at least between voidings. Urine is an easier specimen to obtain and to analyze. It can be readily transported and stored for short periods of time at room temperature, for several days under refrigeration, and indefinitely when frozen. But since the urine concentration of drugs and their metabolites can be affected by time of day, degree of hydration (i.e., how much liquid a person has consumed), exercise (loss of water through perspiration), certain dietary habits, or drugs, it is more difficult to relate any single urine test result to the amount of drug taken or when it was taken. An example of some of these factors is described below.

The choice of analytical method can affect the interpretation of a drug test result. As was previously discussed, an immunoassay result often reflects the concentration of total cross-reacting drugs and/or metabolites. While estimates of such concentrations cannot be related to any one drug species present, many studies have been conducted that show limited relationships between certain assay levels and patterns of drug use. This is described for marijuana below. It should also be recognized that GC/MS or other chromatographic assays usually measure the amount of one drug species. This must be taken into account when comparing results between methods and in published papers. It is necessary to determine what method was used and how the concentration was measured.

Another factor that affects the interpretation of results is the drug itself. Much of this chapter is expressed in generalizations for simplicity. However, there are significant differences between drugs in the way in which they affect people, how they are metabolized and excreted, and in the relative significance of drug test results. It is not possible to present a monograph on each drug here, but the reader should be warned that it takes considerable knowledge of all of these factors and the specific drug in order to interpret drug test results. That is why the federal government requires all test results to be reviewed by a medical review officer. This type of review should be carried out by someone with comparable training.

To give an example of the complexities involved, there follows a brief description of the possible interpretations for positive results for the most commonly encountered drug of abuse, marijuana. Remember that this is a concise and somewhat generalized exposition, so be cautious in applying it to any set of results.

Marijuana

Marijuana and other forms of the cannabis plant produce a wide variety of effects on the human body. Most notable are its intoxicating properties, which usually give the user a desired "high." In general, it also causes variable degrees of impairment of mental and motor functions, such as memory, driving ability, distortion of time and distance, and attentiveness. The magnitude and duration of these effects, which vary widely from person to person, are related to the actual amount of delta-9-tetrahydrocannabinol (THC), the principal psychoactive ingredient in marijuana, absorbed into the body.

The amount of THC entering the system is a combination of the THC content of the marijuana, hashish, etc., and the manner in which it is ingested. Usually, moderate doses of marijuana produce these measurable, but not often noticeable, effects for only a few hours. However, repeated use of the drug over an extended period of time has been linked to longer-lasting effects, such as reduced motivation, possible learning disabilities, depression, and neurological changes. Unfortunately, scientists do not agree on the magnitude of these effects nor on how to measure them.

Modern science, however, has developed methods to detect the presence of and measure the amounts of THC and its metabolic breakdown products in biological specimens, such as blood and urine. These analytical methods have become quite refined and are widely used in the civilian and military sectors to detect the use of marijuana by the testing of urine specimens. Such "urinalysis" can reliably reveal that THC has somehow gotten into a person's body. The questions to be addressed here are how and when did it enter the body, and can the drug test(s) determine any degree of impairment or intoxication, assuming there is some definition of these terms in your own particular company or agency policy.

THC is an extremely fat-soluble chemical. This means that it will not dissolve in water and will be rapidly taken up by fatty tissues in the body. Thus, when marijuana is smoked, the THC is rapidly absorbed through the lung and into the bloodstream, where it is carried bound to blood proteins throughout the body. Once in the blood, THC undergoes two rapid processes at the same time. It is quickly absorbed into almost all tissues in the body, including the brain and heart. It is also rapidly converted in the liver to different chemical forms, known as metabolites. This process is the mechanism by which the body attempts to eliminate foreign substances. Since the metabolites are much more soluble in water, they pass out into the urine where they accumulate until the bladder is emptied.

The process of THC being taken up into body tissues proceeds for about a half an hour, then the reverse occurs. The THC is slowly released back into the blood where it is carried to other tissues and eventually to the liver where it is metabolized and excreted. This continues until all of the THC is eliminated. Of course, if more marijuana is smoked before the first amount is excreted, it adds to that which is stored. There is a "steady state" level that will be reached, however, depending on how much and how often the drug is used.

Scientific studies have shown that THC is eliminated from the body at a rather constant rate. This rate is defined in terms of the amount of time it takes for half the drug in the body to be eliminated. The best estimate for this half-life for THC is 18 to 24 hours (Chiang & Barnett, 1984). This means that half of what was taken in will be gone after one day, 75 percent after two days, 87.5 percent after three days, and so on. This also tells us that if someone smokes one or more "joints" a day, after five days the person will eliminate through the urine the same amount taken in. This is the so-called steady state level. Because frequent or heavy marijuana users take much larger amounts of THC into their body, it will quite naturally take longer for them to eliminate the drug. That is why, in a few cases, users have been found to remain "positive" by the most sensitive tests for as long as eleven weeks (Ellis et al., 1985).

Is there a concentration or range of concentrations of THC metabolite(s) in urine that can be associated with the time of use or with circulating or stored levels of THC in the body, and can such levels be reliably related to any "physiological or psychological effects" of the drug? Studies indicate that a relationship may exist between THC plasma levels and behavioral impairment (Barnett et al., 1985).

The detection of THC metabolites for several weeks, as cited above, was based on the lowest concentration of total metabolites that can be reliably detected in the laboratory. However, many laboratories have established higher detection levels for the initial screening and confirmation tests. Thus, it should be apparent that, with the rapidly falling levels of drug from the body, higher test cutoffs will detect drug use for shorter periods of time. Several studies have shown that it is highly unlikely for a person to remain positive by the 100 ng/mL total metabolite cutoff for more than three days following the use of a moderate amount of marijuana. This use would be detectable for five to seven days at a cutoff of 20 ng/mL. If higher amounts are used, this period of time will be longer. If large amounts of the drug are used daily for more than a week, there is a very small possibility that the person could remain positive at 100 ng/mL for up to a month and for ten weeks at 20 ng/mL.

The second question concerns whether or not these levels can be associated with drug effects. Because the analysis of a single urine specimen cannot distinguish between the two extreme situations cited above, the time of use cannot be assigned with any certainty. However, an elimination of the quantitative urinary levels of the primary THC metabolite, THC-9-carboxylic acid, shows a good correlation with measurable and intoxicating levels of THC in the blood. Thus, concentrations of 100 ng/mL or greater of THC-9-carboxylic acid in urine may be considered as a presumptive indicator (although not definitive evidence) of continued impairment in a majority of cases. Experience has also shown that measurable levels of THC are found in blood specimens collected at the same time as urine specimens containing over 100 ng/mL of the total cannabinoid metabolites over 50 percent of the time.

A frequently heard argument about positive results indicating marijuana use is that the THC got into the person's body through passive inhalation, that is, by inhaling someone else's smoke. Several studies on passive inhalation have been reported to the scientific community in published articles or at national meetings. With the exception of the first report (Zeidenberg et al., 1977), the studies agree as to the possibility of this occurring.

The first report, issued in 1977 by Zeidenberg and colleagues, has been discounted by the scientific community because of the analytical method employed and other problems associated with the study.

The second and most often cited study was conducted by Perez-Reyes and co-workers (1983) at the University of North Carolina. It consisted of three different experimental conditions, one conducted in an automobile and two in a small room (8-by-8-by-10 feet). The levels of exposure varied from two to four cigarettes and, in study 3, on three consecutive days to measure possible cumulative effects. The results showed that only two urines were found positive by EMIT assay. (20 ng/mL cutoff). Semiquantitation of the EMIT results gave concentrations of around 30 to 40 ng/mL equivalents of total urinary metabolites. One of these was quantified by GC/MS, giving 3.9 ng/mL of THC-9-acid. The maximum concentration found in urine specimens collected from the subject from whom blood specimens were taken was found to be 3.0 ng/mL of THC-9-acid.

It should be noted that the conditions necessary to achieve positive results from passive inhalation of marijuana smoke in this series are relatively severe. Of greater significance is that the two positive findings were the first urine voidings, taken at about five hours after exposure. All other studies have shown that peak concentrations are usually found within the first or second urination. As has been pointed out by several experts, it is untenable to suggest that urine samples could be positive by 20 or 100 ng/mL screen and 10 ng/mL confirmation cutoffs beyond twelve, let alone twenty-four, hours after exposure to concentrations of marijuana smoke as generated in these experimental conditions.

There have been several other studies that differ in the levels of exposure and the settings, but they all indicate the same kind of conclusion. It takes a lot of exposure in a small, unventilated space to become positive, even after repeated exposure to marijuana smoke for six days (Cone & Johnson, 1986; Cone et al., 1987). Also, it is important to evaluate the time between any claimed passive exposure and the collection of the specimen when attempting to determine the plausibility of a positive finding having resulted from passive inhalation. Remember that the urine concentration is continually falling, with its frequent ups and downs.

Common Problems

As previously stated, it is essential that every positive drug test result be reviewed by a properly trained person, such as a physician, nurse, or paramedical technician. The provider of the specimen should be asked to explain how the positive finding may have occurred. It will take the judgment of the reviewer as to the plausibility of the explanation, especially in light of the following information and guidelines.

Most drug test results provide proof of illegal drug use. However, there are circumstances with some drugs where an alternate explanation will be offered and may be possible. (This can occur when substances other than illicit drugs have been ingested—either knowingly or unknowingly—by the person being tested.) The following guidelines attempt to cover the most commonly encountered problem areas.

Cocaine

Cocaine is a Schedule 2 Controlled Substance that is still used in certain surgical procedures. In the event of a positive finding for cocaine (usually detected as its primary metabolite benzoylecgonine), surgical procedures could be readily verified.

Two possibilities for unknowing ingestion exist. From time to time, certain herbal teas that contain real coca leaves are imported, mostly into southern California. They are illegal, although this may not be known to the individual at the time. Because of the rarity of finding these teas, strong evidence would be required to determine that this could be a plausible explanation for a positive cocaine result.

It has been demonstrated that as little as 25 mg of cocaine could be placed in a drink, be consumed unknowingly, and produce a positive test result for cocaine for up to two days. Credible witnesses would have to be available to confirm such a claim.

Marijuana

As described in more detail earlier, the psychoactive ingredient in marijuana, tetrahydrocannabinol (THC), is quite fat-soluble and is stored throughout the body. The accepted half-life is about twenty-four hours. Normally, a positive result following the smoking or eating of a "joint" (about 0.5 g) will be obtained for no more than three days. Heavy or frequent use can produce a positive result for up to two weeks. If someone produces a positive result and claims to have smoked just one marijuana cigarette several days earlier, that person is lying. The use was either more recent or a lot more than was claimed.

Passive inhalation of marijuana smoke is possible but highly improbable. At the 100 ng/mL immunoassay cutoff, it would take several days of repeated exposure to the smoke of about thirty cigarettes in an unventilated and small space to produce a positive result. Even under these extreme conditions, quantitative levels of the primary THC metabolite do not exceed 35 ng/mL. Exposure to the smoke of eight joints over one hour under these conditions on six consecutive days never exceed 75 ng/mL of total cross-reacting metabolites (as measured in an immunoassay). Only one of 400 specimens collected exceeded 10 ng/mL on the GC/MS confirmation. It was 12 ng/mL.

It is possible to ingest marijuana that has been cooked into food and to produce positive results for several days (Cone et al., 1988). However, this is unlikely and a credible witness would have to testify as to the nature of the recipe and the quantity of marijuana it contained.

Morphine and Codeine

A positive test for morphine can result from four possible sources. The least likely is pure morphine itself, since it is usually only administered in a hospital. Codeine is metabolized to morphine, so both are usually found following codeine use. This can be verified through the existence of a valid prescription. Usually the codeine level is very high, especially if the use was recent. Occasionally, the level of codeine is less than that of morphine and may be too low to detect, since it is excreted faster than its metabolite morphine. However, the morphine level will be quite low as well.

Heroin is very rapidly metabolized to morphine, which would be found in high concentrations. There is usually some codeine present, since it is a natural constituent of opium and remains as a contaminant in the heroin. It is usually not possible to conclude that someone used heroin in the absence of any other evidence of such use. This would include needle marks or other physiological signs. If heroin use is suspected or if there is no other plausible explanation, the laboratory should be requested to retest the specimen for the presence of 6-monoacetylmorphine, an intermediate metabolite between heroin and morphine. Its presence is conclusive proof of heroin use. A detection level of at least 10 ng/mL is required.

Finally, many poppy seeds that are used in baking are obtained from opium poppies. Depending on their source, some poppy seeds contain sufficient amounts of morphine to produce a positive test result when they are eaten (Fritschi & Prescott, 1985; Hayes et al., 1987). With some of the commercial seeds from Australia and Holland, as little as a tablespoonful can produce a positive morphine result for a day or two. Codeine will usually be present at about 10 percent of the morphine level.

Experience with employment situations indicates that the vast majority of positive morphine and/or codeine results will be due to legitimate codeine use. Care must be taken to determine if there is a valid prescription for the drug. Occasionally, the individual will not remember taking a medication containing codeine or may not have known that it contained codeine. This occurs when the person is given a "pain pill" by a friend or relative. If codeine is ruled out, information about the actual levels found should be obtained from the laboratory. If the morphine and codeine levels are less than 4,000 ng/mL, ask about possible consumption of foods containing poppy seeds. If poppy seeds are ruled out, have the laboratory test for monoacetylmorphine. If it is not present, then it is advisable to give the individual the benefit of the doubt that he or she unknowingly ingested the drug.

Amphetamines

Amphetamine is a relatively small and simple molecule. Because of its close chemical relationship to natural neurotransmitters—the chemicals responsible for many of the body's functions—many drugs are available that are very similar in chemical structure. Some of these are available in over-the-counter cold medications and in diet pills, such as phenpropanolamine (PPA) and ephedrine. Because of the close chemical similarity, many of these drugs may be detected in immunoassay screens, which are designed to detect amphetamine-like drugs. This does not pose any problem when appropriate confirmation methods are used, with one important exception. More specific amphetamine immunoassays are now available.

The two most widely abused amphetamines are dextro- or d-amphetamine (e.g., Dexedrine), racemic or dl-amphetamine (Benzedrine), d-methamphetamine (Methadrine), and dl-methamphetamine. The racemic or dl-forms of these two drugs are usually a product of clandestine laboratories that use phenyl-2-propanone (P2P) as a starting material. The optically active d-forms, which are the most potent isomers, can be diverted from legitimate medical sources or produced illicitly from drugs such as ephedrine or pseudoephedrine. Laboratories conducting GC/MS assays can readily identify these two drugs but have generally not distinguished between the d-, l- or dl-forms.

It has been recognized recently that the overuse of Vicks Inhalers can give rise to the positive identification of methamphetamine in the urine of the user. This results from the fact that Vicks Inhalers contain levo- or l-desoxyephedrine, another chemical name for l-methamphetamine, the weakly active isomer of d-methamphetamine. Concentrations approaching 2000 ng/mL have been seen under experimental and natural conditions. It is now necessary to have laboratories adopt a new assay for confirming amphetamines that makes use of an optically active derivative. The most promising derivatizing reagent is (−)-(trifluoroacetyl)prolyl chloride (TFP). Interpretation of such results can reveal which isomer or isomers were consumed. It must also be recognized that extremely high concentrations of l-methamphetamine can result from abuse of the Vicks Inhalers. It is known that users extract the drug from many inhalers and mainline the residue.

SUMMARY

There has been much loose talk about the accuracy and reliability of drug testing. The news media tend to present half-truths and quotes that are not balanced. The fact is that, when conducted in a rigorously controlled system, which includes strict chain of custody from the time of collection and qualified laboratories, drug testing is highly reliable. It is equally true that there are bad laboratories. This is why it is so important to exercise care and judgment when designing a program and selecting a testing facility. The naysayers would have us believe that drug testing is the culprit, whereas we know that drugs are the enemy. Because it is incumbent on all of us to do what we can to assure a reliable work force, all our efforts should be directed toward keeping out drugs.

APPENDIX   Drug Screening—Laboratory Selection

LABORATORY _____   **FINAL SCORE** _____
                                                       (max 100)

QUALITY OF SERVICES (60 points)
  Test Methods (15 points)   Score _____
  (*Consider sensitivity, established reliability*)
    Screening:

  Confirmation:

Internal Chain of Custody (10 points)   Score _____
(*Consider if description is adequate, methods of identifying
    samples, record keeping*)

Quality Assurance Program (10 points)   Score _____
(*Consider use of standards, internal blind QC, certification of
    standards*)

Turnaround Times, Reporting of Results (5 points)   Score _____
(*Consider how results are reported, timeliness*)

Specimen Collection, transfer to lab (10 points)   Score _____

Provision for Frozen Storage (5 points)   Score _____

Supplies (5 points)   Score _____
(*Consider form design, labeling, security of bottles and kits,
    instructions for use*)

                                 Services Total Score _____
                                                       (max 60)

PERSONNEL (30 points)
  Laboratory Director/Manager (15 points)   Score _____
  (*Consider who will provide expert testimony*)

Management Staff (10 points)   Score _____
(*Is there a full-time toxicologist on the staff and available for
    consultation*)

Technical Staff (5 points)   Score _____

                              Personnel Total Score _____
                                                       (max 30)

APPENDIX   Continued

EXPERIENCE (10 points)
   Licensure/Certification:

   Current Clients:

   Court/Arbitration experience:

                                              Experience Total Score _____
                                                                      (max 10)

GENERAL COMMENTS

REVIEWER _____   DATE _____

REFERENCES

Barnett, G., Licko, V., & Thompson, T. (1985). Behavioral pharmacokinetics of
    marijuana. *Psychopharmacology, 85,* 51–56.
Bowen, O.R. (1988, April 11). *Mandatory guidelines for federal workplace drug
    testing: Final guidelines. Federal Register,* 11970–11989.
Chiang, C.W., & Barnett, G. (1984). Marijuana effect and delta-9-tetrahydrocan-
    nabinol plasma level. *Clinical Pharmacology and Therapeutics, 36,* 234–238.
Cone, E.J., & Johnson, R.E. (1986). Contact highs and urinary cannabinoid ex-
    cretion after passive exposure to marijuana smoke. *Clinical Pharmacology
    and Therapeutics, 40,* 247–256.
Cone, E.J., Johnson, R.E., Darwin, W.D., Yousefnejad, D., Mell, L.D., Paul,
    B.D., & Mitchell, J. (1987). Passive inhalation of marijuana smoke: Uri-
    nalysis and room air levels of delta-9-tetrahydrocannabinol. *Journal of An-
    alytical Toxicology, 11,* 89–96.
Cone, E.J., Johnson, R.E., Paul, B.D., Mell, L.D., & Mitchell, J. (1988). Mari-
    juana-laced brownies: Behavioral effects, physiologic effects and urinalysis
    in humans following ingestion. *Journal of Analytical Toxicology, 12,*
    169–175.
Ellis, G.M., Mann, M.A., Judson, B.A., Schramm, N.T., & Tashchian, A. (1985).
    Excretion patterns of cannabinoid metabolites after last use in a group of
    chronic users. *Clinical Pharmacology and Therapeutics, 38,* 572–578.
Fritschi, G., & Prescott, W.R. (1985). Morphine levels in urine subsequent to
    poppy seed consumption. *Forensic Science International, 27,* 111–117.
Hawks, R.L., & Chiang, C.N. (1986). *Urine testing for drugs of abuse.* NIDA
    Research Monograph No. 73. (DHSS Publication No. ADM 84-1481).

Washington, DC: U.S. Government Printing Office.

Hayes, L.W., Krasselt, W.G., & Mueggler, P.A. (1987). Concentrations of morphine and codeine in serum and urine after ingestion of poppy seeds. *Clinical Chemistry, 33,* 806–808.

Perez-Reyes, M., Di Guiseppi, S., Mason, A.P., & Davis, K.H. (1983). Passive inhalation of marijuana smoke and urinary excretion of cannabinoids. *Clinical Pharmacology and Therapeutics, 34,* 36–41.

Zeidenberg, P., Bourdon, R., & Nahas, G.G. (1977). Marijuana intoxication by passive inhalation: Documentation by detection of urinary metabolites. *American Journal of Psychiatry, 134,* 76–77.

5

Winning the War on Drugs
in the Military

PAUL J. MULLOY

In 1981, I was selected by the Chief of Naval Operations, Admiral Thomas B. Hayward, USN, to lead and coordinate the efforts of many gifted people from the start of the U.S. Navy's drug-abuse initiative. My key objective was to complete this complex and difficult assignment with firmness and compassion. Our watchword was "get rid of the abuse rather than the abusers." The result was that many good people who had gone in harm's way were turned around and today are helping to win our battle against the modern scourge of the civilized world—drug abuse. In sharing this history, I wish to convey my optimism and conviction that good citizens throughout the world can indeed win when each of us gets actively involved. The following is the hands-on account of that story.

In late 1980, the U.S. Department of Defense (DOD) conducted and published a survey of all the armed services on the subject of substance abuse. The survey revealed that marijuana use within the previous thirty days among the E1 to E5 ranks of the essentially 18- to 25-year-old enlisted population was: Army 40 percent, Air Force 20 percent, Navy 47 percent, and Marine Corps 47 percent. Use of any drug (excluding alcohol) by all services was 27 percent (Burt, Biegel, Carnes, & Farley, 1980).

The results were shocking and appalling. They were shocking to senior authorities who lacked knowledge of and sensitivity to the American drug culture's corrosive impact on practices, discipline, and traditional values of young Americans in or out of the military. They were appalling because of the implicit and explicit adverse impact on national security and the combat readiness of its defenders in uniform.

Concurrently, National Institute on Drug Abuse surveys, which had been conducted since 1975 by the University of Michigan, revealed that 67 percent of high school seniors in the United States had used a drug and 37 percent had used marijuana within the past thirty days (Johnston, O'Malley, & Basham, 1986). At that time, for example, the Navy was recruiting approximately 85,000 young people annually from that age base to maintain and build a 560,000-person force.

Many, especially senior officers and enlisted personnel, did not believe the results. The fact that 26 percent of the Navy respondents had reported that they had been "high" on the job made the results even more unbelievable. Subjective responses about alcohol, the number-one drug of abuse, indicated that in the same population over 88 percent had used alcohol and some 21 percent reported loss of on-the-job productivity. Because leaders had greater experience with alcohol-related incidents, they did not question responses about alcohol use.

The focus of this chapter is on the Navy's experience with drug testing because it has been far more extensive than that of the other military arms. However, many of the Navy's experiences and initiatives have been replicated by the other services, by U.S. and foreign governments, and by private industry. Full cooperation and adoption of successful programs between services throughout the early 1980s resulted in varying forms of similar programs. Clearly, the enemy—drugs—remained the same. Programs were designed and implemented to suit the needs of individual services and were supported and supervised by the Secretary of Defense.

EARLY STAGES

Fortunately, urinalysis had been gaining in support both legally and scientifically as a means to detect the presence of licit and illicit substance in the human body. In 1980, the U.S. Military Court of Appeals overturned the 1974 decision *United States* v. *Ruiz* and allowed the use of urinalysis for disciplinary purposes (*U.S.* v. *Ruiz*, 1974; *U.S.* v. *Armstrong*, 1980). This was the critical legal basis for finding no violation of the Fourth (search and seizure) and Fifth (self-incrimination) Amendments applied to military personnel. The court allowed results of a urinalysis as evidence in a judicial and disciplinary proceeding. Technology and laboratory procedures had improved, so that the results were credible. To check the results of the Department of Defense survey, the Navy conducted an anonymous urinalysis survey of its 18- to 25-year-old enlisted population in 1981, which represented about 160,000 individuals. The results slammed home the truth: 47.8 percent of those tested had traces of marijuana metabolite in their urine (Booz, Allen, and Hamilton, 1981). Intense public and political pressure prompted then Secretary of Defense Caspar Weinberger to take action. In the Navy, Secretary John Lehman, Assistant Secretary John Herrington, Chief of Naval Operations (CNO), Thomas Hayward, and the Commandant of the Marine Corps, General John Barrows, authored the following corrective actions that became part of a broader program:

1. Establish a Navy-wide drug prevention education program patterned after the successful Navy Alcohol Safety Actions Program;

2. Strategically place over 200 portable urinalysis kits throughout the Navy and expand urinalysis testing to include tests for marijuana;
3. Test all recruits at the accession point;
4. Increase the number of drug detection dogs from 63 to 200;
5. Expedite placement of ten officer law enforcement positions at major staff locations Navy-wide;
6. Establish drug-enforcement assistance teams on each coast for Master-at-Arms training (Navy law enforcement);
7. Establish an alcohol and drug-abuse management information system to track abuses;
8. Establish Alcohol and Drug Abuse Control Officer positions on all major staffs;
9. Establish drug-abuse education specialist positions at Human Resource Management Centers/Detailments Navy-wide;
10. Establish inspection and assistance teams to improve the drug counseling and treatment effort.

The other military services responded to the pressures and increased resources to expand programs and to add new programs tailored to their own needs and methods.

As these actions were being taken, the Navy was shaken by another event. On May 26, 1981, an aircraft crash occurred at night aboard the aircraft carrier U.S.S. *Nimitz,* killing fourteen people and injuring forty-two others. As tragic as that was, autopsies revealed that cannabis was present in nine of the crew members working on the carrier's flight deck. The pilot of the jet aircraft, a reserve Marine Corps officer who was qualifying for night carrier operations, had been taking a prescribed antihistamine preparation (brompheniramine) without the knowledge of either his commanding officer or his flight surgeon (U.S. Navy Judge Advocate, 1982). This spectacular night crash was aired on nationwide television news shows and reported with misleading but alarming references to drug use by both flight and deck crews. Intensive congressional hearings followed, with demands for corrective action in all services, particularly the Navy and Marine Corps. The crash also resulted in my going to Washington, D.C., to direct actions against drug abuse in the military. To improve the link between technology and policy, the DOD requested Dr. Carlton Turner, the President's Special Adviser on Drug Policy, to convene a conference of nationally recognized toxicologists to examine all aspects of adopting urinalysis in the drug-testing system. All the military services sent their principal line, policy, legal, medical, and technical officers. Technologies, procedures, and policies were developed that would best serve individual service needs while meeting both medical and legal criteria. Advisory boards were established in the DOD and in each of the services. Secretary of Defense Weinberger directed that follow-up surveys be conducted. In addition, the Navy directed that its urinalysis-based surveys would be conducted periodically to assess prevalence and to monitor trends.

Even in the early stages, all services believed that the drug-abuse problem was principally a leadership problem that would require enlightened line leadership to take full responsibility and authority for its solution. To be sure, all clergy, legal, and especially medical personnel were to be intimately involved in proposing and implementing policies, programs, and procedures. Notwithstanding, throughout the process, the line commanders in the chain of command up to the Chiefs of Staff of the Army and the Air Force, the Chief of Naval Operation (CNO), and the Commandant of the Marine Corps clearly assumed full responsibility for resolving this critical readiness issue among uniformed personnel.

Since the Navy was the target of most of the criticism and was under intense scrutiny, many of its plans and programs received the most attention. Several plans were reviewed and eventually incorporated into existing or new programs of the other services. The Air Force Special Action and Army Fitness programs had already been shown to be effective, progressive, and worthy of emulation. The services military branches worked closely together, sharing ideas and information as strategies and tactics were developed to best suit individual service requirements.

Christmas week 1981 was the watershed decision period for the Navy. Parts of the program were coming into place, but the pace wasn't fast enough. The drug issue just wasn't being engaged and resolved in a decisive manner.

GETTING TOUGH

In decisions with the CNO, I recommended that "war" be declared on drugs with all that the phrase clearly implied. I believed that after Vietnam, sailors' values were confused about such things as right/wrong; legal/illegal; traditional beliefs in God, family, and country; and the Navy's customs and traditions. Historically, all these things promoted pride, high morale, and sound discipline. We believed drug usage in the Navy reflected not only a societal malady but also an erosion of our traditional values. Our people needed a clear and unmistakable signal from Navy leadership concerning its resolve, policy, procedures, and objectives.

With the backing of the president and the secretaries of defense and navy, CNO Thomas Hayward provided the signal: unannounced random urinalysis testing of *every* person in the Navy, starting with himself. Testing would also be extended to accidents, inspections, probable-cause incidents, and rehabilitation procedures. All recruits would be informed and would sign an acknowledgment that they would be subjected to urinalysis testing forty-eight hours after reporting to boot camp.

This was a momentous decision, and clearly a courageous and decisive one. Although testing was not the total program, it was a clear signal from Navy leadership of its resolve to use the most effective tool available to rid the Navy of drug abuse. The time of any equivocation had ended. In retrospect, it was the turning point for drug abuse, which had been in-

creasing since the early 1960s in the military, especially in the Navy and
Marine Corps.

The 1980 court decisions had permitted urinalysis testing. What authorized the CNO to act was a memo from the Secretary of Defense in
December 1981 to all military branches rescinding any prohibitions on the
use of urinalysis as evidence in disciplinary proceedings, including in administrative discharges (Secretary of Defense, 1981). Based on this ruling,
the military commenced testing in 1982, but the Navy's program was
clearly the most aggressive and ambitious of any. If it was to succeed it
had to have solid backing from the White House and the administration—
which the CNO got.

The CNO's decision for extensive testing came about after intensive
discussions concerning obstacles, logistic hurdles, and budget limitations.
Shortages of laboratory personnel and others trained in testing were analyzed, as were the uncertainties about collection procedures and the potential for human error. We knew this was brand new ground. The risks
were evident but the stakes were high. All shortcomings were accepted
because throughout the "war on drugs," in any of the procedures, in any
of the processes, in any of the evidence, one of the cardinal underlying
principles I insisted upon was: "Where there is doubt, throw it out." In
other words, if there is any doubt—not just legal "reasonable" doubt,"
decide in favor of the individual. The reason for this policy was obvious:
the Navy's deterrence strategy was not going to be compromised by the
acknowledged errors that would be made in getting drug testing fully on
line. The consequences to an individual reputation and career were too
severe. We wanted to change attitudes and behavior, and so, as previously mentioned, the guiding principle became "get rid of the abuse, not
the abuser." Help would be provided to any member of the Navy,
whether officer or enlisted personnel, who sought help in a non-manipu-
lative way. The help would be professional, and immunity from prosecution would be guaranteed unless manipulation was involved. This was a
critical policy decision to turn peer pressure around and get the majority
to work for a drug-free military and against pushers and recalcitrant users.
The policy of "zero tolerance" was clear! The penalty for disobedience
was severe: For officers guilty of one-time drug use, dismissal from the
service under less than honorable conditions; for enlisted personnel, who
were the vast majority, the granting of one more chance. The commanding
officer (CO) could offer a second chance if he believed the individual's
performance, otherwise, and potential showed promise for productive
service.

Of great and reassuring satisfaction was the decision made about our
chief petty officers (CPOs), the traditional backbone of the Navy. Some
thought they too should receive a second chance. I suggested taking a
sounding with our Master Chief Petty Officer, the number-one enlisted
man in the Navy. He surveyed CPOs around the fleet and came back with
a resounding recommendation: "No! One time out!" As with the officers,

the basis was clear: their trusted positions of leadership-by-example required immediate discharge for drug use. Traditions formed at sea and in combat for "the leadership trinity of authority, responsibility, and accountability" were reaffirmed in that one decision.

IMPLEMENTATION

During the discussions there were some who wanted to delay implementation of random urine testing. But it was decided that the urgency of the situation would be further demonstrated by rapid implementation of a nononsense policy. Thus, February 1, 1982, was declared D Day for commencing both random and other forms of testing in the war on drugs. Some were very skeptical of the decision, but others were less concerned because of the inviolate condition of "any doubt—throw it out," which would preserve the presumption of innocence on the part of those who tested positive for drugs. Errors were anticipated because of the sheer size and complexity of the undertaking and, especially, its newness. Accountability for correcting the anticipated mistakes was personally stressed by the CNO and later was dramatically validated by actions taken on behalf of individuals when the system did err. Nothing like this had ever before been done on such a scale. From its original role in medical treatment, urinalysis became a major all-Navy readiness tool. With an ultimate objective of testing everyone three times a year, requiring 1.8 million specimens and 10.8 million tests, one remark described it aptly: "We're going to issue hip boots to the laboratory people as the tank cars of urine roll in!"

The Commandant of the Marine Corps was simultaneously conducting similar planning sessions, and both the Navy and Marine Corps headquarters staff worked closely in formulating policies and procedures. Assistant Secretary John Herrington (later Secretary of Energy in the Reagan administration) supervised all planning for Secretary of Navy Lehman, who was responsible for both the Navy and the Marine Corps.

An important parallel to the efforts against drug use was an equally strong message against alcohol abuse. We were vulnerable to charges of double standards and hypocrisy if we didn't engage the issue of excess use of the number 1 drug, alcohol. Therefore, we began to get tough on alcohol abuse by changing traditional "wetting down" practices and other customs that had in the past encouraged the rite of passage through overindulgence. Alternatives were promoted. "Happy Hours" would remain because they encouraged unit cohesion and personnel camaraderie for combat readiness, but the excess use of alcohol was discouraged. The "your booze, my grass" charge was engaged. Alcohol abuse gradually declined, although admittedly the measures were not as vigorous as the anti-drug initiatives.

The 1981 Christmas decision to implement widespread testing encompassed many other intiatives, which became a blueprint for subsequent successful programs in both the military and civilian sectors in this country. These have been used as well in other countries, which are now feeling the effects of illicit drugs. Thus the blueprint had many facets.

Based on credible and verified assessments provided by the surveys, a multi-program implementation plan was initiated. It included provisions to inform all hands, from admirals and generals to seamen and privates, of the policy and how it was to be implemented. All communications—from briefings, to print, to television and radio broadcasts, to every ship and station—were started in January 1982. In keeping with the enlightened leadership premise, briefings were conducted in San Diego, California, Norfolk, Virginia, and Washington, D.C., to all admirals and generals who were available to attend. An analogy in private industry would be division-level briefings of corporate and company executives. Full-day presentations of legal, medical, security, counseling, treatment, and disciplinary issues, problems, and solutions were given by experts in each field, and also by those officers responsible for conducting the overall program. Special emphasis was placed on the urinalysis testing program and the nature and extent of drug abuse.

Perhaps here it should be stressed that we knew we were dealing with twin obstacles: denial ("Drugs can't possibly be in my outfit") and ignorance among the more senior, older officers, CPOs, and NCOs. From their experience in Vietnam and at sea, many had some idea of drugs and the effects of drug use, but they lacked insight gained from scientific, professional, and rehabilitative perspectives. That learning process had to begin and be sustained in order to provide sure knowledge for competent leadership. It was replicated thereafter by the briefing of each senior attendee throughout his subordinate command organizations around the world.

Simultaneously, messages that clearly spelled out the policy and the provisions were drafted and released by the Secretary of the Navy, the CNO, and the Commandant of the Marine Corps. The management principle of having leadership communicate to all who would be affected by the new policy—a strategy essential to the program's success—was implemented.

Internally, the Navy formed a task group of senior action officers representing line, legal, public relations, medical, and chaplain corps to monitor actions taken and to advise with regard to initiatives or corrective steps. This group coordinated with similar entities in each of the military branches, as well as with the Drug Policy Board established by the Assistant Secretary of Defense for Health Affairs.

The flag/general officer briefings provided direct feedback to policy and program formulation at the meetings and, more importantly, the mechanism for fleet feedback, which exists even today for a "howgozit" on the "war on drugs." The two-way flow was an important provision because, in fact, there were differences of abuse, drug type, and availability between the Atlantic and Pacific fleets and overseas bases. In like manner, the experience of the Air Force and Army varied by country. For example, hashish was of concern to commanders in the Mediterranean littoral and in Germany, but not to those on the West Coast of the United States, where amphetamines were a major concern.

METHODOLOGY

For all the services, 1982 was an especially intensive year. Administration and congressional pressure for solutions to the drug problem and rapid progress was intense. Congressional budget hearings in February accentuated the need for action. The White House Drug Scientific/Technical Board had gathered some eighteen biochemists, toxicologists, and experts in related fields to assist the DOD in formulating correct technological procedures for processing and testing urine specimens. Expert guidance was provided on testing equipment and methods, the critical issue of minimum levels, and standards for laboratories and techniques. Potential problems, such as an individual testing positive for marijuana by exposure through passive inhalation, were explored thoroughly. In the end, driven by leadership/management objectives, a standard was reached about acceptable scientific parameters to initiate and sustain the urinalysis testing program safely and soundly. Throughout the early years, this board of experts was available to leadership and management for technical and scientific advice.

At the Department of Defense, the Drug Policy Board, composed of flag officers, general officers, and senior civilians, and chaired by the Assistant Secretary of Defense (ASD) with the direction and assistance of the White House Drug Policy Advisor, provided policy and procedure guidance to the individual services, as well as standardized policy and doctrine for the whole Defense Department.

To implement drug testing, each service proceeded at a different pace and scope. The Navy, along with the Marine Corps, went all out on urinalysis testing and multiple programs. The survey assessments provided baseline information on prevalence and the urgency of the drug problem. Understandable concern was expressed by senior officials in the Office of the Secretary of Defense that the Navy was proceeding too quickly. If testing failed, it could decimate the military services and the entire initiative could be lost in the courts. Also, there were the very real uncertainties about widespread urine collection, chain of custody, laboratory capabilities and limitations, legal minefields, and other unknowns.

These concerns were also shared by some in the Navy. However, the decision to declare a "war on drugs," in light of the widespread prevalence of drug use, brought the most effective component—to test extensively—up front in a balanced multiprogram effort. The obstacles and potential for scuttling hazards cannot be overemphasized. Urinalysis testing was an enormous undertaking with a relatively short start-up time considering the available resources for processing specimens.

In January 1982, nine laboratories were available to the DOD to conduct urinalysis. The Army had three, located in Wiesbaden, Germany; Fort Meade, near Washington, D.C.; and Trippler Army Hospital in the Hawaiian Islands. The Air Force had its large lab at Brooke Air Force Base in Texas. The Navy (which also provides medical support for the Marine Corps) had four laboratories: in San Diego and Oakland, California; in Norfolk, Virginia; and in Jacksonville, Florida.

Prior to the introduction of widespread testing, urinalysis had been essentially limited to the medical requirements of the associated hospitals, which average about 350 specimens per month per laboratory. By 1983, the Navy's program would require analysis of 30,000 specimens per month at each existing laboratory and the opening of a new facility at Great Lakes Naval Station near Chicago, Illinois, as well as contracting for a civilian laboratory. The other services had similarly geared up for their increased urinalysis processing.

A rigorous "standard operating procedure" was developed for each element of the testing program, with corrections and modifications applied as experience dictated. What eventually evolved became a model for procedures in many federal and corporate programs worldwide. There are very few scars that the system hasn't endured in the learning process that haven't been put to the benefit of other subsequent initiators. The Navy's plan was to test all personnel three times yearly for six substances: cannabis, cocaine, barbiturates, amphetamines, PCP (angel dust, phencyclidine), and opiates. Since 1983, about 10 million tests have been processed annually.

To ensure accuracy in the laboratory, a two-tier system of verification was dictated. Screening of all specimens would be conducted by one process: Either radioimmunoassay or any other immunoassay or approved procedure. Minimum levels recommended by the White House and approved by the Secretary of Defense were established. For example, 100 nanograms per milliliter (ng/mL) was the standard cannabis detection level. Any specimen above 100 ng/mL was considered a presumptive positive and was then subjected to a confirmation process. Initially, only gas chromatography, and later gas chromatography/mass spectrometry (GC/MS), was required for confirmation. This state-of-the-art equipment to perform these tests was made available to all laboratories. A more difficult provision was to locate and hire technically competent operators in sufficient numbers.

Confirmation levels for each substance were established also by the Secretary of Defense. For example, 20 ng/mL was required for cannabis. The concern about passive inhalation on the part of the person being tested was eliminated by adhering to that level after screening at the 100 ng/mL level. If a specimen was found to be positive, the specimen was frozen and retained in controlled custody for one year. This enabled any defendant to have the substance available for retest in any legal proceedings. Subsequent judicial rulings have supported these procedures, and similar requirements are in the 1988 "Federal Guidelines for Testing and Laboratories."

It is important to explain here that in determining the 100 ng/mL screening cutoff and cutoffs for other substances, a key element in the policy was more than determining just presence of the illicit substance. The objective was to identify the chronic or addicted user. A minimum level of 100 ng/mL for cannabis, the most extensive illicit drug of abuse, was expected to identify nearly 60 percent of users, only the current high users. For the rest of the users, it was hoped that screening would motivate them to change their behavior. In particular, I hoped that, with time, the majority peers of nonusers would influence the others. Above all, a sense of fairness coupled with firmness, rather than trickery or terrorism, had to prevail. The elements of the fourth and fifth amendments were upheld also in this approach. The fear of losing so many people (48 percent identified in the 1981 survey) with trace amounts of cannabis in the all-volunteer military services was mollified. The goal wasn't just to catch users; it was to help them become reliable members of the military. It worked. During that critical first year less than 1 percent were discharged!

Mistakes were made in implementation. Attempts to control the volume of flow to the laboratories while they were increasing personnel and equipment were insufficient. By mid-1982, the system was showing cracks. Distribution to one laboratory was suspended; another was shut down when its administrative and operating procedures were found to be in violation of the standards. Quality-control procedures, inspections, safeguards, and review procedures had been imposed. When the system erred, the safeguards detected the shortcomings. When several thousand specimens at one laboratory were mishandled, the operation there was stopped, an ad hoc review board was formed, and over a period of several months over 42,000 records were reviewed. More than 8,000 individual records were reinstated, 80 percent of these had positive laboratory confirmations of substance abuse, but the results had to be ignored because handling procedures had been violated. These violations included errors in collection, chain of custody, and laboratory procedures, as well as incorrect Social Security numbers, and mistakes in individual names. The principle remained: "any doubt, throw it out." Any discrepancy was ruled in favor of the individual. As painful and time-consuming as that experience was, it probably ensured the program's success. The results were published and credibility and trust in the system was established. By 1983, the Navy's drug-screening program was operating satisfactorily.

SAFEGUARDS

One of the greatest challenges was the staffing of laboratories. The earliest priority was the locating and hiring of qualified GC/MS supervisor/

operators. After that equipment, maintenance, and physical and personnel security systems and procedures were addressed.

To maintain quality control, various external and internal safeguards were established. The Armed Forces Institute of Pathology (AFIP) in Washington, D.C., was directed to institute a system for proficiency testing. Thirty-six samples per week (70 percent negative and 30 percent positive) are sent through field activities, ashore and at sea, to each laboratory. The laboratory does not know these are quality-control specimens. Additionally, 24 samples known to be controls are sent directly to each laboratory from AFIP each month. Eighty percent of these contain traces of known substances and 20 percent are negative. Furthermore, inspection teams from the DOD, CNO, and offices of the surgeon general of the Navy and of the other services conduct frequent visits to their laboratories to review all aspects of the program, including qualifications, security, chain of custody, confidentiality, and administrative details. Moreover over 20 percent of all specimens tested annually in the labs are retested as an internal quality-control measure.

Of great pride and reassurance is that since 1982, with over *48,000 known negative* samples processed, *zero false positives* (that is, negative samples being called positive) have been identified in the Navy system. Considering that over 80 million tests have been conducted, this is a significant fail-safe element in the system.

To give the reader an idea of the magnitude of annual testing, a comparison between 1985 and 1986 (see Table 5.1) shows the increases in urinalysis specimens tested (*Military Drug and Alcohol Program Report,* 1987):

TABLE 5.1　Number of Specimens Tested Annually

	1985	1986	Percent Increase
Army	692,149	765,505	10.6
Navy/USMC	1,463,480	1,938,534	32.5
Air Force	183,984	207,864	13.0

At the time of this writing, each Navy/USMC specimen is tested for seven substances; each Army and Air Force specimen is tested for two.

Perhaps one of the most important safeguards is the final step in processing a positive finding from the laboratory. In addition to the requirement that the laboratories be accurate, reliable, and confidential was the mandate that *the laboratory is never the judge.* Because the drug issue was conceived to be a leadership issue, the final step was the commanding officer's judgment. The laboratory's determination of the presence and level of an illicit substance could be reaffirmed, but the commanding officer had to satisfy himself by any means and beyond any doubt that the person accused had "knowingly and willingly ingested the substance."

Current directives have reaffirmed the role of the CO, ruled against judgments based solely on laboratory findings, and acknowledged that instances of innocence, accident, and malice could occur.

Actual instances of marijuana-spiked cookies and other spiked drinks and food did occur. Careful investigation and in-depth interviewing of acquaintances of the people involved precluded unjust action against them. The objective of zero tolerance with deterrence and detection was strengthened by the review process. Even after a guilty finding, further review steps, including a board at the CNO level, were available to all contenders. Similar procedures were instituted in each service to maintain confidence and system credibility.

WINNING THE WAR

Random testing was the most controversial, difficult, and potentially vulnerable program put into effect in the war on drugs. Without question, it has been successful. As applied, it has sustained repeated court examinations and repeated and extensive evaluations. Wherever mistakes are made, each individual case is reviewed and reversed if doubt exists. In 1983, a private research firm was hired to conduct an independent survey to determine the effectiveness of the many programs implemented in the war on drugs. The population previously surveyed (which had the greatest numbers of offenders) was queried. Eighty-three percent of the respondents said that the number-one deterrent was random drug testing. Perhaps even more significantly, 28 percent stated that if it weren't for testing, they would still be taking drugs (Booz, Allen, & Hamilton, 1983)!

When testing hit its stride, many young people made comments like: "It's about time"; "the dogs and the [urinalysis test] kits mean you're serious." One comment that reflects the power of peer pressure for the casual or occasional user or experimenter, which is equally applicable today and in industry, is, "Now, I have an excuse to say no."

There are two key aspects of any successful drug-testing program. One is specimen collection and the other is chain of custody. Both require strict, accountable procedures. The weakest link is the collection procedure. It should be conducted as methodically as any procedure that could result in disciplinary discharge and legal action. Chain of custody starts when the specimen is delivered to the container in the presence of a witness. Experience has shown that offenders will resort to any method to circumvent positive findings: adulteration, substitution, and dilution. Therefore, the observer must be mature, responsible, and trustworthy.

The Navy's program has experienced shortcomings in these areas. Some senior enlisted personnel have been court martialed for complicity in attempts to thwart the system. Without compromising the requirement for a witness, the settings, clothing, and conditions of the actual collection require privacy and respect for the individual's dignity to the extent actual field or shipboard conditions permit. Observers must be of the same sex. In other professions and occupations where direct observation is not permitted, such as with current federal guidelines for civilian employees, rigorous restrictions must be imposed to preclude such fraud as: water bluing, no access to hot water, use of gowns, temperature-sensing devices, etc.

Chain-of-custody procedures are equally rigorous. They include sealing of the container with tamperproof material; initialing by the donor, the observer, and the collection official; and administrative entries on permanent record sheets. These all accompany sealed shipping containers, which are sent directly to the laboratories, usually by U.S. mail. An important provision for confidentiality is to use bar-code or Social Security numbers in place of the name of the donor to identify his or her specimen throughout the processing steps. A reverse procedure occurs at the laboratory, where individual reading, labeling, and content of each specimen are strictly maintained. All aspects of the system are randomly inspected for adherence to procedures.

Weapons Used in the Drug War

A major initiative that took place early in the drug war was the fleet's introduction of urinalysis test kits and drug detecting dogs. Because deterrence was the principal objective, both kits and dogs were visible proof of the intent, resolve, and ubiquitous presence throughout the Navy.

The kits resulted from a request to industry to provide a rapid means to identify abusers. A key factor was accident/incident prevention, such as with sailors who might be handling weapons, steering a ship, operating vehicles or equipment, or performing any number of the myriad complex and hazardous daily duties in the modern Navy. Responding to the challenge, SYVA Co. of Palo Alto, California provided a kit called EMIT S/T (single test), which is portable, can test for six drugs, takes only ninety seconds to determine drug presence, and is accurate initially at the 95 percent or better level (now, around 99 percent). For deterrence and prevention until full delivery systems were provided, six hundred kits were obtained. They were superb, and SYVA provided the technical teams to ensure operator competence and proficiency. To be sure, the results could only be considered *presumptive* positive and *not* used for legal or disciplinary procedures. In the event of a positive finding for drugs, no punitive action or conclusion could be based on kit results alone. However, the offender could be removed from any hazardous duty that could affect his or her personal safety or that of shipmates. Elaborate testing, recording, and transmittal procedures were followed to maximize confidentiality and chain of custody. A positive specimen would be entered into the system to receive a separate screening (immunoassay and confirmation GC/MS) test in the laboratory. The kits have been a major asset in the drug-testing program. Even today, in remote, hazardous, or high-security areas, they are an excellent tool in the drug-prevention war. SYVA also produced high-volume equipment and reagents, which are used extensively and reliably in the field and laboratories—a good example of industry meeting national security needs.

Drug-detection dogs were also needed and represented a roving symbol of deterrence. Trained as a team, operators and dogs (close to three hundred in number) were assigned to major combatant ships (all aircraft carriers and major task forces), as well as to major stations worldwide. Frequently, one would see a dog and handler passed from ship to ship by traditional Navy highline, and the crew knew what was up. Small dogs, like beagles, were preferred because they avoided a "gestapo" image, and also for practical purposes: they could crawl into inaccessible places, under deck plates and behind bulkheads, and could be lifted up to inspect overhead piping. Try doing the latter with a reluctant Doberman! An ancillary result was that the dogs became mascots that the crew protected from mischief or harm. The animals also provided another positive image to encourage intensifying peer pressure against those involved with drugs.

The kits and dogs were effective deterrents. One could joke that even a kit that didn't work and a dog with a cold nose would keep most drugs from coming on board ship just by being at the gangplank. Nevertheless, the Navy was constantly challenged by the ingenuity of the American sailor who was bent on obtaining drugs. For example, in the beginning of testing, baby urine in San Diego was selling for $50 a container. "Specimens" of bourbon, engine oil, and jet fuel have also been collected. The current temperature-sensing devices for urine specimens were a response to such substitution tricks. These and other precautions are particularly important where direct observation is not required or allowed.

Concomitant with these major programs, all the military services expanded morale, welfare and recreation activities, family facilities, and fitness programs, and they initiated substantial improvements in training, education, and treatment. Knowledge and alternatives, along with testing, were key components of the offensive against drugs.

In the Navy an appeal was made successfully in 1982 in congressional hearings not only to retain the fledgling Family Service Centers (FSCs) but also to expand them globally. Full briefings and tours were conducted to counter the resistance both externally and internally to this novel but vital concept. With 82,000 sailors at sea at any given moment, it was believed that care and assistance to dependent families was an important aspect to the substance-abuse effort. The FSCs provided a locus for information, assistance, education, budget, and nutritional guidance for newly married spouses, and they would be a link to the counseling and assistance network for spouse, child, and substance abusers. Eventually, eighty-three centers were established worldwide, and the Navy was acclaimed by *Money* magazine as one of the "Ten Terrific Employers" in the nation (*Money* magazine, 1985).

Another major effort promoted physical fitness as a part of combat readiness and as an alternative to substance abuse. An entire fitness regimen was established at every command with required standards of performance. Additional funds were obtained to expand existing gymnasia and related facilities, add modern equipment and supplies, and build new facilities. Major additions were provided to ships for at-sea use. The emphasis on physical fitness served well as an alternative to substance abuse and to relieve stress. It also contributed to the concept of "getting high on oneself." This was one area in which all services made major advances, with the Army, especially, providing the initiatives. Fitness programs should be a key consideration for deterring drug abuse in any industry.

Without question, one of the most expansive improvements was in the field of education. In addition to the measures already mentioned, the Navy established a thirty-six-hour advanced training school called NADSAP (Navy Alcohol, Drug, Substance Abuse Program). It consists of thirty-six hours of formal, intensive education on substances abused; their sources, effects, symptoms, and treatment; leadership skills; attitude and values clarification; coping and communication skills; and alternatives for healthier lifestyles. Junior and middle-grade officers, as well as senior petty officers, attend this course, which is conducted by professionals contracted from the University of Arizona. Over 50,000 personnel attend each year in over one hundred "classrooms" worldwide. A one-day course is also available for command managers and supervisors whose schedules do not permit attendance at the full-week course. Coupled with mandatory formal education for recruits and fleet personnel, "vincible ignorance" is being eliminated.

The following are some of the data for cost analyses of all these programs established to win the war on drugs. For all branches of the military services, drug and alcohol prevention programs cost $214 million in fiscal year 1986, as compared with $172 million in fiscal year 1985 (*Military Drug and Alcohol Program Report,* 1987). Accounting procedures were responsible for the principal increase. Monies expanded in 1986 for drug testing are listed in Table 5.2.

Available Navy statistics demonstrate a commitment to increase drug/alcohol funding (Table 5.3). In FY 1981, $26 million was allocated, of which 81.2 percent was expended on treatment, 10.8 percent on prevention, and 8.8 percent other. In FY 1985, $81.7 million was spent, of which 47.9 percent went for prevention activities, 46.8 percent for treatment, and 10.2 percent for training, evaluation, planning, and research. The le-

TABLE 5.2   Cost of Drug Testing in 1986 (in U.S. dollars)

Army	18,588,000
Navy	30,540,000
Air Force	2,492,000
Marine Corps	775,000
Total	52,395,000

TABLE 5.3 Navy's Expenditures for Drug and Alcohol Programs
(in millions of dollars)

	Treatment	Prevention	Other	Total
1981	21.1 (81.2%)	2.8 (10.8%)	2.3 (8.8%)	26.0
1985	38.2 (46.8%)	39.1 (47.9%)	8.3 (10.2%)	81.7

gal decision that permitted urinalysis, combined with the military's prior emphasis on alcohol awareness and with new leadership, brought about this major budgetary shift (Interview with Captain Leo A. Canginelli, 1988).

A cost-benefit analysis of treatment revealed that in FY 1985 7,378 people were treated at a cost of $20.6 million with 80 percent success (2-year follow-up data). When analyzed in terms of cost to replace, the Navy saved about $169.2 million in recruitment, training, and experience (which meant higher pay and allowances) of a senior petty officer. Less certain were the monies saved by preventing accidents and injuries caused by drug use. For example, the estimated replacement cost for aircraft destroyed or damaged as a result of the *Nimitz* crash was over $53 million. Other benefits have been the high retention and combat readiness of personnel, strengthened leadership and discipline, and improved morale. As Owens-Corning Ford Co. observed: for every dollar utilized in Employment Assistance Programs, [it] gets back $9.00 (Interview with G. Bunn, 1988).

To provide the help promised to those who seek and need it, all services have expanded counseling, assistance, and treatment facilities and capabilities. The Navy established a three-level system. Level I has individual Drug and Alcohol Program Advisers for every unit, ship, squadron, station, and base. They provide preventive education and aftercare (very important follow-up), urinalysis, and self-referral (help with immunity) conducted by individual command counselors. Level II Counseling and Assistance Centers (CCACs) are located at major Navy installations around the world, plus twelve at sea on aircraft carriers and task forces. At these centers, screening, counseling, and family assistance are provided by Navy counselors. Over 28,000 people utilized CCACs in 1987. Today, eighty CCACS are in operation worldwide. The most extensive help is available through Level III professionally staffed treatment centers, Alcohol Rehabilitation Centers (ARCs), and the Alcohol Rehabilitation Departments (ARDs) in Navy hospitals. These centers offer six- to eight-week residential treatment programs. Counseling, individual therapy, group therapy, education, and family counseling are provided by medical personnel and credentialed Navy counselors. The four major centers include the facility at Long Beach, California, which helped Betty Ford and Billy Carter with their drug dependencies. The centers have superb success records.

The treatment centers have been supplemented by more than two dozen Alcohol Rehabilitation Departments at Navy hospitals, which also treat patients with other drug dependencies. Unique to the Navy among all the armed forces is its 196-bed Drug Rehabilitation Center at Miramar Naval Air Station, California. In the early years, it provided drug-specific treatment and gained knowledge of the world of the drug culture from the victims themselves. Many of the lessons learned have been applied directly to the entire deterrence/detection system. The center has since been expanded to treat patients with alcoholism and eating disorders.

In waging the war on drugs, a major effort was expansion of training and education. The levels of ignorance and interest varied from the young recruits to the senior officers and enlisted personnel. Courses and materials were prepared to span that rather wide culture spread and to convey the full spectrum of information on the problems and the programs being initiated. Subjects included lists of illicit substances; their sources, appearances, and effects; policies and programs; assistance and treatment; legal and security measures; values clarification; and leadership skills.

Print and, especially, video media were employed extensively worldwide on every Navy ship and station. All aspects of the war on drugs were presented, from personal messages from the CNO and others directing the program to descriptions of the equipment, laboratories, legal procedures, available treatment, and the illicit substances themselves. It was the most extensively covered topic ever conducted in the Navy's media history. A memorable clip features Chief of Naval Operations Admiral Hayward with the, "Not on my watch, not on my ship, not in my Navy" message. With steely but compassionate eyes, his message was clear: "If you need help, we will help you; if you continue to violate the law and hazard our shipmates, we will hammer you." It left no doubt in the minds of every sailor—from admiral to seaman!

Recreational facilities were expanded substantially to include games and educational video offerings and to provide personnel with further alternatives to drugs, especially during quiet hours at sea or on bases.

COUNTERING DRUG TRAFFICKING

Drug trafficking has been a major concern for the military, especially trafficking through the U.S. mails. Whereas the Army and Air Force could call on Federal Postal Inspectors for assistance, the Navy could not when its ships were at sea or at remote stations. The Navy sought congressional help to resolve the massive abuse of U.S. mails by traffickers, who were immune from prosecution because of postal regulations that barred the opening of packages by anyone other than the intended recipients themselves. This was evident when boxes containing illicit drugs broke open in a ship's mailroom, but the ship's captain was prohibited from taking action because of the postal ban. Another time the British Customs official on the island of Diego Garcia in the Indian Ocean could open suspicious U.S. mail but the U.S. Navy captain standing beside him could not. Congressman Glenn English (D-Okla.), Chairman of the Government Operations Subcommittee and a staunch advocate of anti-drug measures, after hearing of these incidents, gave the DOD and U.S. Postal Service thirty days to correct the problem for all the military branches. It was done. Henceforth, where postal inspectors were not available overseas or at sea, commanding officers could authorize the inspection and confiscation of mail or packages suspected of containing contraband, and prosecution could follow. The change in regulations was widely publicized and a major conduit was closed off to drug traffickers.

Another important improvement in security was the hiring of additional agents for the Naval Investigative Service. These agents operate worldwide, coordinating with other law enforcement agencies in the United States and in foreign countries. They also conduct undercover operations aboard ships and at naval stations. They are a critical arm in the war against the most sophisticated criminals the Free World has encountered.

RESULTS

The military has seen the positive benefits of its many programs and concerted efforts against alcohol and drug abuse. For all military services, the use of *any* drug over the past thirty days decreased from 27 percent in 1980 to 8.9 percent in 1985 (*Military Drug and Alcohol Program Report,* 1987), and this downward trend continues today. Loss of productivity due to alcohol decreased from 34.4 percent in 1982 to 27.1 percent in 1985, again with a continuing downward trend. In the Navy, where testing is most extensive, success has been the score. Since 1982, all performance records have improved and fewer than 1 percent of Navy personnel have been discharged. Urine samples positive for marijuana declined from 48 percent to 21 percent in the first year of testing, to under 10 percent in the next year, to about 2 percent in 1988 (Department of Defense [DOD] Survey, 1988). Since 1982, the Navy's laboratories have had no false-positive results from 48,000 blind negative samples. Where administrative errors did occur, the review and appellate process corrected them. When translated into corporate language of profit and a competitive edge, the advantages of an enlightened substance-abuse program are apparent.

Ever since 1986, the federal government has mounted a major effort to formulate rules, instructions, and guidelines for civilians employed by the government. Agents of the Justice Department, FBI, Secret Service, Drug Enforcement Agency, and Customs Service were among the first civilian employees to be tested. Testing of new recruits began in the summer of 1986. Since mid-1987, the Customs Service and the FBI have been testing their agents randomly, and the Department of Transportation has introduced testing at nine of its ten agencies, including the FAA, FRA, and Urban Mass Transit. The FAA has already subjected 19,000 air traffic controllers to random testing. Thirty-three thousand who are in sensitive positions are subject to random urinalysis testing. The Coast Guard and the Secret Service also have full programs of testing, including random urinalysis.

The Department of Health and Human Services (DHHS, responsible for federal guidelines) has published a document titled "Technical and Scientific Guidelines and Laboratory Control Standards" that outlines procedural guidelines for the drug testing of forty-seven federal agencies, representing 95 percent of the total federal work force, including civilian employees in sensitive positions and those involving public safety. Direct observation of specimen collection has been prohibited by Executive Order except when an employee has violated the normal conditions of collection. Laboratories involved will be subjected to rigorous quality-control measures patterned after the proven military laboratory standards and operating procedures. The DHHS "Guidelines" provide the specific requirements for testing and the laboratories. In the private sector, the Department of Transportation issued its final ruling on 1 December 1989, which imposed drug testing on about four million workers, ranging from airline pilots to teachers in safety-sensitive positions.

After conducting four major regional meetings around the country, the White House Conference for a Drug Free America held its concluding conference in March 1988, in Washington. The president, key cabinet members, and congressional leaders made impassioned pleas to expand the war on drugs. Widespread testing—including random testing—was warmly supported, especially for government posts in which public safety and national security are involved. Even union representatives in attendance favored pre-employment and for-cause testing, although they strongly resisted random testing of union members on grounds of rights of privacy and personal dignity. Even so, participants and attendees were expected to recommend to the president that drug testing be extended. During his successful campaign for the presidency George Bush vigorously supported these recommendations.

Global concern is growing. Support for drug testing among American citizens and outrage against criminal drug activity are on the rise. Even European military units have initiated testing in response to the rise in drug abuse. The trend is clear. Testing is being recognized as a credible and viable deterrent when other means just don't do the job.

Key lessons can be learned from the military experience. The program described here, which consists of ten elements, can be adopted, in whole or in part, by others in government or private industry.

An effective program should consist of the following:

1. Assessment of problem and attitude among employees and environment
2. Formulation of policy specific to the organization

3. Policy and program communication
4. Education and training
5. Counseling, treatment, and rehabilitation (Employee Assistance)
6. Security improvements
7. External support
8. Substance abuse alternatives
9. Drug testing
10. Quality assurance

To gain maximum employee willingness, I strongly recommend that these ten points be implemented incrementally. Thus, one could begin the assessment phase with surveys, focus groups, and individual interviews to determine attitude, behavior, and drug prevalence unique to the culture. Look at the Ten Point program as a scope through which to focus and approach a company or community problem.

With the preliminary assessment and optimum employee involvement, develop a policy. Develop each point separately over time so that the persons testing (randomly), if involved, will likely have gained strong employee support for a drug-testing program.

I have used this approach successfully with clients. Of course, pre-employment testing should be adopted early to protect workers from bringing drug users into the workplace and also to prevent charges of negligent hiring. The program works as a deterrent, a detector, a cost-avoidance tool, and a performance-enhancement system.

As described elsewhere in this book, courts have come to support policies that include testing when the need is evident and individual safeguards are assured. The concepts and programs cited here have served as models not only for the federal government and corporations but also for foreign governments and their military services and private companies. Testing, including random testing, should be an integral part of any plan to curb drug abuse, and it should be available when other programs don't succeed. In the Navy, it was the number-one deterrent. The programs cited were effective because they are people oriented and principle oriented. They have been designed to deter, but they can detect and punish as required. They are affordable because their costs are offset by the gains in productivity. The alternative is clearly unacceptable.

Winning the war on drugs is not only possible, as shown by the experiences of the U.S. military, but it is a must, and the only option available for a free society.

ACKNOWLEDGMENTS

I acknowledge and commend the many dedicated leaders in our armed services, government, and private industry who made this pioneering program against drugs so effective. Their intelligence, perseverance, and pursuit of excellence contributed to formulating, enacting, and perfecting the most successful and oldest counter-substance-abuse program in the world. Its ten essential points described herein have formed the basis of programs adapted by other agencies of the U.S. government, foreign governments, corporations, and small businesses with which I have worked for so many years.

REFERENCES

Booz, Allen & Hamilton, Inc. (1981). Urinalysis test results analysis (survey). Arlington, VA.

Booz, Allen & Hamilton, Inc. (1985). Relative effectiveness and impact of Navy drug control initiatives. Arlington, VA.

Burt, M.R., Biegel, M.M., Carnes, Y., & Farley, E.C. (1980). Worldwide highlight from the Worldwide Survey of Non-Medical Drug Use and Alcohol Use Among Military Personnel: 1980, Bethesda, MD: Burt Associates, pp. 6–7.

Department of the Navy OPNAV Instruction 5350.4A of 27 August 1987, *Alcohol and Drug Abuse Prevention.*

Interview with Captain Leo A. Canginelli, U.S. Navy. Drug and Alcohol Prevention and Control Program; Office of the Chief of Naval Operations, March 17, 1988.

Interview with G. Bunn, Director, Employee Assistance Programs, Owens-Corning Ford, at White House Conference on Drug Free America, March 2, 1988.

Johnston, L.D., O'Malley, P.M., & Basham, J. G. (1986) "National trends in drug use and related factors among American high school students and young adults, 1975–1986, Rockville, MD: Department of Health and Human Services.

Military Drug and Alcohol Program Report (FY 1986) prepared by the Office of the Assistant Secretary of Defense for Health Affairs, April 1987.

"Ten terrific employers." (1988, May).*Money* magazine.

Presidential Executive Order 12564, of September 15, 1986, in *Drug free federal workplace.*

Secretary of Defense, Memorandum for Secretaries of the Military Departments, Directors of Defense Agencies. Subj: Alcohol and Drug Abuse, dated December 28, 1981, signed by DEPSECDEF Frank Carlucci. (Rescinded all prior memos/rules and authorized use of urinalysis for disciplinary reason.)

U.S. v. Ruiz, 23 U.S.C.M.A. 181, 48 CMR 797 (1974); *U.S. v. Armstrong,* 9 M.J. 374 (1980).

U.S. Navy Judge Advocate General investigation and report. Final endorsement (11th) from the Secretary of the Navy. June 29, 1982.

6

Drug Testing in Athletics

ERIC D. ZEMPER

Attempts to control drug use by athletes through drug testing and education have increased considerably in recent years, as has the amount of public attention to the use of drugs by athletes. This chapter will present some of the background concerning drug testing in athletics, particularly with regard to the author's own experience with intercollegiate athletics. The philosophical considerations behind the rationale for drug testing in an athletic context will be discussed, as well as an overview of legal concerns as they apply to athletic drug testing. Finally, the current status of athletic drug testing will be presented, along with a look at possible future developments.

It should be kept in mind that a number of factors make drug testing in athletics unique in comparison with drug testing in the workplace, the military, or elsewhere. While non-athletic drug testing generally has focused on illegal drugs that hinder work performance, drug testing in athletics has focused primarily on legal drugs that are taken to artificially enhance athletic performance. (As will be pointed out, the emphasis on illegal drugs in athletic drug testing is a very recent phenomenon.) Except for testing done by the federal government on employees or military personnel, non-athletic drug testing generally has been done on a local level, while most athletic drug testing has involved national or international sports-governing bodies. Finally, athletic drug testing primarily has focused on a class of drugs never considered in non-athletic drug testing: the anabolic steroids. This latter fact has a number of implications for testing protocols, the timing of testing, the type of equipment, and the expertise required of the personnel doing the testing. But like drug testing in non-athletic settings, the testing of athletes raises a number of philosophical and legal questions, some of which can be addressed in a straightforward manner and many of which, as we shall see, still present no clear-cut answers.

It also should be kept in mind that drug testing of athletes must be one aspect of a comprehensive total program of education, testing, and treatment, as is the case with many athletic testing programs, particularly in collegiate athletics. However, this chapter will focus only on tne testing of athletes.

BACKGROUND

Brief History of Drug Testing in Athletics

The initial development of drug testing for athletes was spurred in the early 1960s by the death of a European cyclist at the 1960 Olympic Games who had been using amphetamines in an attempt to improve his performance. The Medical Commission of the International Olympic Committee (IOC) began development of a drug-testing program that was first implemented on a preliminary basis during the 1968 Olympic Games in Mexico City, and then began the first comprehensive testing at an international competition during the 1972 Olympic Games in Munich. Testing was done for amphetamines and other psychomotor stimulants that had the potential to enhance athletic performance. During the 1976 Olympic Games in Montreal, after an accurate test had been developed, the IOC also began testing for anabolic steroids (Catlin, 1987).

Throughout the 1970s and the 1980s the IOC has been the leading organization in athletic drug testing, developing the testing protocols and specimen-handling procedures, and funding research on improving testing methodologies. The IOC has certified and monitors a network of drug-testing laboratories throughout the world, currently numbering nineteen, that must meet rigid criteria for quality and accuracy of their testing procedures. In addition to a thorough on-site review of each laboratory's facilities, staff, experience, written testing protocols, quality-control measures and reference standards on hand, the IOC Medical Commission also submits a series of ten urine samples containing known drugs or combinations of drugs (or possibly no drugs). All test samples must be identified and properly documented with 100 percent accuracy within three days. An IOC-certified laboratory undergoes recertification on a yearly basis, and undergoes proficiency testing twice a year.

The IOC Medical Commission also has developed a very precise and detailed protocol for collecting, identifying, handling, and transporting urine samples from the time athletes are selected for testing until testing is completed, to avoid misidentification of samples and to eliminate the possibility of successful legal challenges based on mishandling of samples. In recent years the IOC drug-testing protocols and methodologies have served as the basis for the development of testing programs for the major sports-governing bodies in the United States, such as the U.S. Olympic Committee and the National Collegiate Athletic Association (NCAA). The current list of drugs banned by the IOC includes over a hundred substances in six different categories that could be used to artificially enhance an athlete's performance (see Table 6.1). This list is continuously reviewed and modified as new drugs in the six major perfor-

TABLE 6.1 Substances and Methods Banned by the International Olympic Committee

I. *Doping Classes with Examples*

A. Psychomotor stimulants, e.g.:
  amphetamine
  benzamphetamine
  chlorphentermine
  cocaine
  diethylpropion
  dimethylamphetamine
  ethylamphetamine
  fencamfamin
  meclofenoxate
  methylamphetamine
  methylphenidate
  norpseudoephedrine
  pemoline
  phendimetrazine
  phenmetrazine
  phentermine
  pipradol
  prolintane
      and related compounds

B. Sympathomimetic amines, e.g.:
  chlorprenaline
  ephedrine
  etafederine
  isoetharine
  isoprenaline
  methoxyphenamine
  methylephedrine and related
      compounds

C. Miscellaneous central nervous system
      stimulants, e.g.:
  amiphenzole
  bemigride
  caffeine[a]
  cropropamide
  crotethamide
  doxapram
  ethamivan
  leptazol
  nikethamide
  picrotoxine
  strychnine
      and related compounds

  codeine
  dextromoramide
  dihydrocodeine
  dipipanone
  ethylmorphine
  heroin
  hydrocodone
  hydromorphone
  levorphanol
  methadone
  morphine
  oxomorphone
  pentazocine
  pethidine
  phenazocine
  piminodine
  thebacon
  trimeperidine
      and related compounds

E. Anabolic steroids, e.g.:
  bolasterone
  boldenone
  clostebol
  dehydrochlormethyl-testosterone
  fluoxymesterone
  mesterolone
  methandienone
  methenolone
  methandrostenolone
  methyltestosterone
  nandrolone
  norethandrolone
  oxandrolone
  oxymesterone
  oxymetholone
  stanozolol
  testosterone[b]
      and related compounds

F. Beta-blockers,[c] e.g.:
  acebutolol
  alprenolol
  atenolol
  labetalol

(continued)

[a]If the concentration in the urine exceeds 12 μg/mL. (At least 8 cups of strong coffee are needed at one sitting to reach this level.)
[b]If the ratio of the total concentration of testosterone to that of epitestosterone in the urine exceeds 6.
[c]Tested for only in specified sports; e.g., archery, shooting, figure skating compulsory event.

TABLE 6.1 Continued

D. Narcotic analgesics, e.g.:
  anileridine
  metoprolol   bumetanide
  nadolol   canrenone
  oxprenolol   chlormerodrin
  pindolol   chlortalidone
  propranolol   diclofenamide
  sotalol   ethacrynic acid
  timolol   furosemide
      and related compounds   hydrochlorothiazide
G. Diuretics, e.g.:   mersalyl
  acetazolamide   spironolactone
  amiloride   triamterene
  bendroflumethiazide   and related compounds
  benzthiazide

II. *Doping Methods*

A. Blood doping
B. Pharmacological, chemical, and physical manipulation of the urine

III. *Classes of Drugs Subject to Certain Restrictions*

A. Alcohol
B. Local anesthetics
C. Corticosteroids
D. Human chorionic gonadotropin

mance-enhancing categories become available, and in response to attempts by the athletes to circumvent the testing procedures.

Historically, the primary purpose of drug testing of athletes has been to ensure fair competition by discouraging the use of performance-enhancing drugs. The essence of sport has always been competition between athletes based on their individually developed natural abilities, not on the basis of who can find the most effective chemicals. But in a society that is increasingly drug-conscious and has given ever-greater accolades to "winners," it seems inevitable that many athletes will turn to the use of drugs in order to win.

Performance-enhancing drugs fall into two major categories: psychomotor stimulants and anabolic steroids. Psychomotor stimulants, such as amphetamines, cocaine, ephedrine, and caffeine, act in a variety of ways to enhance the functioning of the central nervous system, which in some cases can translate to better athletic performance. To enhance athletic performance, these drugs must be taken immediately prior to the competition and, because they stay in the body a relatively brief time, any testing for them must occur soon after the competition in order for the drugs to be detectable.

Anabolic steroids are used to increase muscle bulk and strength (and therefore, to some extent, speed), and to enhance recovery from heavy workouts or certain kinds of muscular injuries. In some sports, such as football or the weight events in track and field, the increased muscle bulk and strength translates to better performances on the athletic field. To enhance athletic performance, anabolic steroids must be taken over a long period of time (weeks or months), well before any competition. In contrast to psychomotor stimulants, anabolic steroids tend to stay in the body for relatively long periods, making their detection much less dependent on testing immediately after use.

Also banned is the use of narcotic analgesics because of their ability to mask pain, which may lead to more serious injury, and because of their addictive nature. For certain sports, primarily archery and rifle or pistol marksmanship, drugs that act to depress the nervous system or slow heart action, and therefore allow steadier aim at a target, can act as performance enhancers. Competitors in these sports, therefore, are tested for alcohol and other depressants, and for beta blockers, which slow the heart rate. One additional category of drugs tested for is diuretics. There are two reasons for testing for these drugs. First, diuretics sometimes are used (and abused) in an effort to lose weight quickly in sports where athletes are categorized by weight, such as wrestling and weightlifting. Second, they often have been used to dilute the urine in an attempt to mask the presence of other banned drugs.

Testing for the so-called recreational drugs or street drugs has never been a concern of the IOC and other international sports-governing bodies for the simple reason that these substances are not performance-enhancing drugs. The exceptions to this generalization are amphetamines and cocaine, which are psychomotor stimulants, and therefore are among the drugs tested for by the IOC. Street drugs such as marijuana, LSD, or PCP generally have no potential to enhance athletic performance and, in most cases, will act to inhibit athletic performance. Because these drugs cannot be used to gain an unfair competitive advantage, they have never been included in the testing programs of the IOC and other international sports organizations.

In the United States, however, in recent years much of the drug-testing activity in sports has been directed at street drugs. The roots of this emphasis in the United States can be traced to the recent intense media coverage of the drug problems of American society in general and in professional sports in particular. The appearance in 1982 of an article in *Sports Illustrated* by former professional football player Don Reese was among the early events that for the first time began to focus public attention on the problem of drug use in sports (Reese & Underwood, 1982), despite the fact that there had for many years been growing concern in athletic circles about the increasing use of performance-enhancing drugs. The big difference was that Reese was a star in a major professional sport and the problem was street drugs, which was something the general public could relate to much more easily than to some shot-putters using anabolic steroids. The publicity surrounding the disqualifications of several athletes at the 1983 Pan American Games in Caracas, Venezuela, and the sudden departure of a number of U.S. track and field athletes before they had competed and could be tested served to convince the public that the drug problem was not limited to professional sports or a few obscure amateur athletes.

The cocaine-related deaths of college basketball player Len Bias and professional football player Don Rogers a few days apart in 1986 further galvanized public opinion. These events occurred just as the NCAA and several of its member colleges and universities were beginning to implement drug-testing programs for their athletes, and the U.S. Olympic Committee was well into implementing its new drug-testing program, which was developed in response to the Pan American Games incident. Because of increasing media coverage of the street-drug problem in America and the rapidly growing number of reports of street-drug use by professional athletes, there developed a public perception that there was a "major drug problem" (i.e., street drugs) in all of athletics. Naturally, there was a public outcry to do something about it.

As this public sentiment was growing, many colleges and universities, noting the bad publicity that professional sports were receiving, realized that college athletics would be the next focus of media attention, with the attendant impact on relations with state legislators, alumni donors, and the general public. There was a strong feeling within the college ranks that the drug problem among college athletes was not as great as it seemed to be in professional sports, but something still needed to be done to head off this problem. The most obvious and visible solution for some schools was to test athletes for drugs. It would demonstrate that the great majority of college athletes were "clean," and those who were not could receive appropriate help. Many schools also began drug-education programs for their athletes instead of, or in combination with, testing. Professional sports were unwilling or unable to pursue this approach because of objections from a number of professional athletes, backed by strong unions. In 1983–84 a small number of colleges and universities began drug-testing programs for their athletes. All of these programs tested for street drugs; almost none tested for anabolic steroids.

In early 1984, at the request of its membership, the NCAA assembled a panel of experts in athletic drug testing to make recommendations concerning a national testing program.* Technically, according to NCAA "protocol," the committee makes its *recommendations,* which then serve as a basis for the development of a proposal (by the NCAA legislative services staff), which is then voted on by the membership at the annual convention. This panel submitted its recommendations for a program based on the IOC testing program and the newly implemented U.S. Olym-

---

*During the period 1982–1985 the author was the NCAA Research Coordinator. At this time, he was staff liaison to the expert committee and was responsible for writing the recommendations and technical protocol developed by that committee.

pic Committee plan. Among the specific recommendations was that the NCAA test only for performance-enhancing drugs, because of the legal complications inherent in a national sports-governing body testing for illegal street drugs that have no positive impact on athletic performance and, therefore, are outside its reasonable responsibility to ensure fair competition. Because of a number of administrative and communication problems in trying to get the proposed drug-testing plan ready for approval by the membership at its annual convention, the original plan was tabled for further development at the NCAA convention in early 1985. A new drug-testing committee, composed primarily of coaches and athletic administrators, was formed to complete development of an acceptable plan. The new committee started with the plan recommended by the previous panel as a basis, but made an immediate major change to include street drugs in the testing program. The new plan was adopted in early 1986, and the first testing was done during NCAA championship events and post-season football bowl games of the fall season of 1986.

In 1984 the NCAA Drug Education Committee began surveying the NCAA membership about the existence of drug education and drug-testing programs at member schools. Of the nearly one hundred institutions that indicated they had in place or were planning a drug-testing program for their athletes, all were testing for street drugs and less than one-quarter indicated they were testing for the primary performance-enhancing drugs, anabolic steroids. It was apparent that the NCAA membership was not following the established logic of testing only for drugs related to athletic performance but was taking on the unrelated task of testing for street drugs in response to the public outcry to do something about the perceived street-drug problem in sports. This occurred even though there was no evidence whatsoever that the street-drug problem in college sports was any greater than in the general population in that age group. This was a major move away from the historical purpose of drug testing in sports.

Philosophical Issues

At this time, let us focus on the issue of performance-enhancing drugs, leaving aside the issue of pleasure-enhancing drugs for the moment. There is little question that in recent years the use of performance-enhancing drugs has become a growing problem in athletic competition. With the increasing infatuation of the American public with sports, fed by the print and electronic media, and America's penchant for glorifying winners, winning "at any cost" gradually has become the accepted and even expected norm. Add the powerful impetus of national pride and the political and philosophical differences between the Western nations and the Eastern bloc countries, which tend to get translated into international sports competition (i.e., the dubious premise that "our country's athletes did better than your country's athletes, therefore our country and our political system are superior"), and it is no longer surprising that many athletes are constantly pursuing an elusive "competitive edge," no matter what the risk. For many athletes this pursuit extends to the point of being willing to risk health or life by taking dangerous drugs in order to be a winner. There has to be concern about the priorities of athletes who admit, as many did in a recent poll of top-level athletes, that they would opt to take a drug that would greatly improve their chances of winning an Olympic gold medal even though such a choice would carry with it a high probability of causing their death within four years. There also has to be serious concern about the priorities of a society that pushes athletes to this state.

As observed by Murray (1983, 1986), many athletes are put in an extremely coercive situation in which they feel they must use performance-enhancing drugs. Because of society's extreme emphasis on always being a winner, and the strong suspicion that athletes from other countries are using drugs, many American athletes feel they are under a great deal of pressure, from coaches or fans or from their own extremely competitive natures, to use performance-enhancing drugs rather than be at a perceived competitive disadvantage. Many athletes have stated that they do not want to use drugs but feel they have no choice if they want to have any chance of competing well against those they believe are using drugs. Individuals with the potential ability and the desire to be outstanding athletes should not be placed in such a coercive situation.

Much of the discussion in athletic circles about whether or not athletes should use performance-enhancing drugs in order to compete on an equal level with those who do use drugs tends to ignore the one basic fact about the use of these substances. In the simplest of terms: It is cheating. There is no denying that the use of any performance-enhancing drug is contrary to the basic spirit and intent of athletic competition; it distorts the very nature of sport. The competition should be decided on the basis of who has done the best job of perfecting and utilizing his or her natural abilities, not on the basis of who has the best pharmacist.

If the use of performance-enhancing drugs in sports is so widespread, and other athletes feel they must use them to compete successfully, why not drop the prohibition against these drugs and let everyone use them? That would certainly eliminate the need for testing, with all of its attendant problems and costs, and everyone would then presumably be on an equal footing again in competition. The answer to this argument is complex, involving a number of medical, ethical, and philosophical considerations. It basically comes down partly to health and safety considerations, but primarily it is a question of whether or not the basic nature of sport should be maintained or drastically changed.

Certainly an important reason not to drop the prohibitions against performance-enhancing drugs involves the long-term health and safety of the athlete. Here we are considering primarily the use of anabolic steroids, the major class of drugs used by athletes to improve performance, although, as noted at the beginning of this chapter, the use of psychomotor stimulants also has its dangers. The use of anabolic steroids, particularly the extremely large dosages used by athletes, carries with it a great risk of a number of adverse side effects, ranging from mild to deadly. Among the milder side effects are acne, premature baldness, prostate enlargement and inflammation, increased aggressiveness, testicular atrophy, and reduced sperm production. In adolescents, the use of anabolic steroids causes premature closure of the growth centers of long bones. Thus, such individuals will not be as tall as they would have been had they not used the drug. In females, anabolic steroid use results in side effects such as masculinization, abnormal menstrual cycles, and irreversible changes such as excessive body and facial hair, enlargement of the clitoris, and deepening of the voice.

At this time it is difficult to be precise about many of the side effects, because experience has shown that exposure to some drugs does not result in the appearance of side effects until as many as fifteen to twenty years later. However, it is becoming clear that some of the more dangerous long-term side effects of anabolic steroid use include psychoses, kidney dysfunction, liver disease, including cancer, and alterations in serum lipid profiles that indicate an increased risk of cardiovascular disease and heart attacks. In recent years there has been a small but growing number of documented deaths of young athletes attributed to anabolic steroid use, primarily among power lifters and body-builders, the sports that have the longest history of steroid use. Considerations of the long-term health and safety of the athlete therefore are important reasons for continuing the ban on the use of these substances.

While it might be argued that an athlete should be free to choose whether or not to take such "individual" risks, this argument is an over-simplification of the situation. Such a decision is not made in a complete vacuum; the decision by one athlete to take such a risk to improve performances does not affect that athlete alone. Any other athlete this person competes against is then placed in the coercive situation of either choosing also to take the risk to his or her health by using the drugs or choosing to compete at a disadvantage. A talented athlete should not be forced to make such a decision about participating in an athletic competition.

Most importantly, however, dropping the ban on performance-enhancing drugs in sport would also entail a major revision of the nature of competition. Athletic competition traditionally has been between individuals or groups of individuals based on the development and skillful use of their bodies and their natural abilities. It is known that drugs such as anabolic steroids react differently in different bodies. Some individuals may gain a great deal of strength from the use of the drugs, while others may gain very little. Therefore, the use of these substances by all athletes would introduce a new element into sport: the innate ability of the body to respond to the drugs (Fraleigh, 1985). So, another basic argument for continued ban of these substances is that sport should be a competition between *individuals,* based on the development and utilization of their natural physical and mental skills; it should not be reduced to an assessment of the ability of their bodies to benefit from the ingestion of drugs.

Legal Implications

Until recently, the legal issues involved in drug testing in sports were not very complex. Testing was done only for banned performance-enhancing drugs rather than illegal street drugs. The International Olympic Committee and other sports-governing bodies tested only at closed competitions where agreeing to be tested was a condition of entry into the competition. These very restrictive parameters for drug testing generally caused few legal problems, even in the United States, where constitutional provisions regarding such legal concerns as privacy and due process are much stronger than in most other nations of the world. American courts generally recognized that participation in sports was a privilege rather than a right, and sports-governing bodies had a legitimate interest in ensuring fair competition by testing athletes to see that they were not using banned performance-enhancing drugs. Such testing was quite well established and accepted.

In recent years, however, the situation has changed considerably with the decision of the National Collegiate Athletic Association and its member colleges and universities to include in their new drug-testing programs the unrelated category of illegal street drugs, and with the attempts to test for street drugs in some professional sports. This has opened the collegiate drug-testing programs to a number of legal challenges, as evidenced by a continuing series of court cases involving the NCAA and several of its members who had implemented local drug-testing programs for athletes. The primary rationale that has been developed for including street drugs involves concern for the health and safety of the athlete. It is argued that health and safety will be compromised if athletes participate in arduous practices or competitions while under the influence, say, of a drug like marijuana. The safety of teammates and competitors also could be adversely affected by the participation of an athlete using drugs. While such a rationale appears somewhat reasonable, it has not been tested in the courts. It also needs to be backed up with solid evidence of such short-term harm to the health and safety of the athlete.

One recent legal development concerning the NCAA, outside the realm of drug testing, may have an impact in the future. In 1989 the U.S. Supreme Court decided in favor of the NCAA in a case involving NCAA sanctions against the University of Nevada-Las Vegas basketball coach Jerry Tarkanian for violation of a number of NCAA regulations. An important element in this decision was the Supreme Court's affirmation that the NCAA is a private organization and not a "state actor" or extension of a government entity, even though a large number of its membership are colleges and universities supported by state governments, and therefore they could be considered "state actors." As a private organization, the NCAA is not subject to some of the more stringent constitutional and legal requirements regarding due process and equal protection, to which governmental entities are subject. This principle that the NCAA is not a "state actor" had generally been accepted by lower courts in recent years with regard to legal challenges to NCAA regulations and procedures, but it had not been completely confirmed by the highest court. With the affirmation of this principle by the Supreme Court in the Tarkanian case, it no doubt will be easier for the NCAA in the future to defend its drug-testing program in the courts with regard to legal challenges based on constitutional due process and equal protection requirements.

At the time of this writing, several cases are being tried and several others have been decided in the lower courts, with the NCAA and its member schools winning some of them and losing others, and with all of them in various stages of appeal. It is difficult to pick any single case that is representative of all, since most cases involve different testing programs developed locally at each school and usually involve differing sets of laws that often are unique to the particular state or community where the case is being tried. It is very likely that this entire issue eventually will be settled by the Supreme Court.

It appears from some of the lower-court decisions that there has been a lack of a clear distinction between testing for street drugs and testing for performance-enhancing drugs in sports. This distinction also appears to have been unclear to many college and university athletic administrators as they attempted to respond to public concern about drug use in sports. In the courtroom and elsewhere, such a lack of clarity in distinguishing between these two separate types of drug testing carries with it an immediate danger to the established principles of testing for performance-enhancing drugs in sports. If the courts ultimately decide that the NCAA and its members cannot test their athletes for drugs because of the legal problems inherent in testing for street drugs (outlined elsewhere in this book), in a "worst case" situation this also could include prohibition of testing for *any* drugs, including performance-enhancing ones.

Such a result would have major implications for American athletes in international competition. In international sport circles, the United States already is seen as a "foot dragger" with regard to drug testing of athletes, because many foreign sports officials do not fully understand the extent of the protections provided by our Constitution and our legal system, and why we therefore must be so cautious about implementing drug-testing programs. While the rationale of the NCAA and its members for including street drugs in their testing programs needs to be tested in the courts, the failure to maintain a clear distinction between testing athletes for street drugs and testing for performance-enhancing drugs could endanger the current ability of sports-governing bodies in this country to test for performance-enhancing drugs.

The Problem of Anabolic Steroids

With the possible exception of *professional* athletes, it has been found that street drug and alcohol use among athletes is no greater than among the general population of the same age. The primary drug-use problem that is unique to athletes is the use of anabolic steroids, to which we will now turn our attention.

Over the last thirty years there has been a great deal of disagreement as to whether or not the use of anabolic steroids actually does improve athletic performance. This argument has continued ever since anabolic steroids first were used by power lifters and body-builders in the late 1950s and early 1960s. In the early 1960s the practice spread to the weight-event athletes in track and field, who shared weight-room facilities with power lifters and body-builders, and eventually to athletes in other sports. On the one hand, athletes and their coaches are convinced anabolic steroids can do wonders, and on the other hand, most of the medical and scientific community point to the fact that there is essentially no research data supporting such claims. The athletes' claims are based primarily on locker room testimonials and other anecdotal data. The few published research studies supporting their position have not been accepted by the scientific community because the studies have been poorly designed. The scientific and medical community pointed out that the use of anabolic steroids caused the body to retain fluids, which probably accounted for much of the weight gain seen by those who use these substances. In addition, studies showed that there appeared to be a strong placebo effect involved. Athletes who thought they were receiving anabolic steroids but who were given inactive drugs gained as much strength and weight as those who actually were given anabolic steroids. In other words, athletes who take anabolic steroids *expect* to gain strength, and therefore train harder in anticipation of that effect, thus creating a self-fulfilling prophecy.

While the research literature leaves little doubt that anabolic steroids can increase the muscle mass of castrated animals or the strength of a sex-related muscle in rats, there is no generally accepted research showing any effects in increasing muscle mass or strength in intact humans. The major problem with doing research in this area is that no human-subjects review committee would allow a study on humans using the massive doses of anabolic steroids used by athletes. The medically recommended dosages of anabolic steroids range from 2.5 mg to 10 mg per day; athletes use 100 mg to 400 mg per day. Therefore, there has been no practical way to complete well-controlled experimental studies to test the athletes' claims. These huge daily doses of anabolic steroids are the reason for the concern about the health of athletes using these drugs, as mentioned earlier. We know of several deleterious side effects from the use of a few weeks' course of the recommended medical dosage of these substances, but at this time no one knows for sure what the long-term impact on health will be from months or years of taking the huge doses used by some athletes. Results from the few studies that currently are becoming available are raising legitimate concerns, but we are still a long way from being able to specify what the probability of various side effects will be for use of different amounts of all the many different anabolic steroids.

Added to this is the problem of the general unwillingness of most athletes to discuss details of their use of anabolic steroids, making it difficult even to estimate the prevalence of usage.

The major difference of opinion regarding the efficacy of anabolic steroids has resulted in the medical community losing a great deal of credibility with the athletes and coaches. The medical community has followed its usual conservative procedures by maintaining the position that no definitive proof exists that use of anabolic steroids increases muscle mass or strength in normal, healthy humans, since there are no well-designed scientific studies to support such a claim. However, the athletes believe such a position is ridiculous when they feel they can see all the proof they need every day in the weight room. As a result of this lack of credibility, the medical community now is finding it difficult to convince the athletes of the reality of the dangerous side effects of anabolic steroid use that currently are being documented. Recently, some members of the medical community that work most closely with athletes have come to the conclusion, based on a growing amount of indirect evidence, that anabolic steroids can increase muscle mass and therefore strength in some individuals, but the evidence also indicates that the effect varies greatly from one person to another. Some individuals appear to make significant gains, while others gain very little.

In addition to not believing the medical community regarding the lack of scientific proof that anabolic steroids work, many athletes are skeptical of the claim that testing for these drugs cannot be circumvented. Ever since drug testing of athletes began in earnest more than twenty years ago, and particularly since testing for anabolic steroids began in the mid-1970s, there has developed a kind of vicious circle of competition between the athletes who feel they have to use drugs and the sports authorities who are trying to eliminate performance-enhancing drugs in sports. As soon as testing began, athletes started looking for ways to circumvent the tests. As they became successful in doing so, the testers began developing more extensive testing programs and more sophisticated methods to counteract the attempts at circumvention, which in turn led to further attempts by the athletes to find undetectable drugs or ways to mask the drugs. This cycle continues today, with each side seeking ever-more sophisticated ways to stay one step ahead of the other.

The various types of attempts by athletes to circumvent the testing procedures generally can be broken down into three categories: substitution methods, masking methods, and use of drugs or methods that currently are not detectable. The least sophisticated category is the attempt to avoid providing the athlete's own urine through various means of substitution. These methods were predominant during the early years of athletic drug testing, and included such ploys as hiding a balloon or other container of another person's urine on the athlete's person and emptying it into the collection container during the specimen-collection procedure, or catheterizing the athlete and introducing another person's urine into the athlete's bladder prior to testing. These methods led to the now legendary joke in athletic circles that "his test results showed no traces of anabolic steroids, but he's three months pregnant." The "balloon method" was made essentially impossible by the adoption of stricter protocols requiring the provision of the urine sample under direct observation by a drug-testing team member. The "catheterization method" was made essentially useless with increased sensitivity of the testing equipment. Even though most of the urine specimen of the "catheterized" athlete is from a "clean" person (i.e., someone who has not used the drugs for which the tests are being conducted), there still will be a certain percentage of the specimen that will be the athlete's own urine containing the drug. The urine can be concentrated in the laboratory and the traces will be picked up by the testing equipment.

The second circumvention category is through various means of "masking" the presence of the drug. The earliest and crudest attempts were simply diluting the urine sample by adding water from a toilet bowl while providing the specimen. This ploy was countered by placing a blue dye in the toilet bowls in the specimen-collection area and by the requirement of direct observation of the person providing the specimen. More sophisticated approaches include the use of drugs like diuretics to dilute the urine, or probenecid, to inhibit the excretion of urine. These methods are countered by the increased sensitivity of the testing equipment, and by including such drugs on the list of banned substances.

The third category of circumvention is use of drugs or methods that currently are not detectable. These include human growth hormone, erythropoietin (an experimental drug that only stays in the body a few days, but which causes the production of increased amounts of red blood cells, whose oxygen-carrying capacity is critical in endurance sports), and "blood doping," or withdrawal of an amount of blood from an athlete, storing it, and reinfusing it just prior to a competition, after the body has replaced the withdrawn blood, thus providing increased numbers of red blood cells. Tests for human growth hormone and blood doping are being developed, and they already have been placed on the IOC/USOC (United States Olympic Committee) list of banned drugs and doping procedures. Erythropoietin is very new, very expensive, and is not yet available except in small amounts for laboratory use, but the IOC Medical Commission will no doubt be giving this drug very careful consideration in the near future.

Part of the reason why this "competition" continues between the athletes and the drug testers is the complexity of testing for anabolic steroids. There are at least twenty different anabolic steroids available, which is enough of a problem to begin with. Add to that the fact that one does not look for the anabolic steroids themselves in the urine being tested, but rather for all of the metabolites or metabolic breakdown products of the steroid that are excreted in the urine. Each steroid compound can have as many as a dozen or more metabolites. It is a very complex process to sort out and identify all of the varied metabolites of an anabolic steroid compound from among all the other metabolites the body normally produces. If the athlete has been "stacking," or taking two or more different anabolic steroids at once, as is often the case, the task becomes even more complicated.

This task is made possible by use of gas chromatography and mass spectrometry (GC/MS) testing equipment. GC is used initially, and any specimens showing indications of an illicit drug are then put through the mass spectrometer, which operates at a molecular level to identify compounds present in the specimen. In addition to complex and expensive equipment, the entire process requires very skilled lab technicians with a great deal of experience in identifying the metabolites, but when properly done it is essentially 100 percent accurate. However, very few labs are capable of doing completely accurate tests for anabolic steroids. While many labs may have the appropriate GC/MS equipment, most do not have the personnel with the extensive experience necessary to identify the complex spectra of metabolites of anabolic steroids. The complexity of the process and the need for complete accuracy is why the IOC has set such rigid standards for certification of drug-testing facilities. But the complexity of testing for anabolic steroids also opens the possibility of trying to circumvent the detection of the drugs by using other agents to alter the pattern of metabolites in the urine or slow their excretion rate to undetectable levels, or by finding new, slightly altered anabolic steroid compounds that have not yet been characterized as to their metabolite pattern by the testing labs and thus could essentially be "invisible" to the testing procedures.

Another problem with testing for anabolic steroids is the fact that they do not have to be used immediately prior to competition to gain benefit from their use, as is the case with psychomotor stimulants. Until now, testing has been done only at major national and international competitions, so athletes essentially have been free to use the drugs during their training and then stop use a few weeks before the competition to allow time for the metabolites of the drug to be cleared from the body. This is the major reason testing has not been as effective in stopping the use of anabolic steroids as it has with psychomotor stimulants.

Most people involved with drug testing in sports agree that the only effective way to test for anabolic steroids is to have random, unannounced tests throughout the year, which would give the athlete using the drugs no chance to clear his or her body of traces of the drug before being tested. The national sports federation in Norway has used this procedure for several years to test its athletes, no matter where in the world they may be residing or training. Proposals to do unannounced testing have been considered by the IOC and other international sports-governing bodies, such as the International Amateur Athletics Federation (track and field), and by some U.S. sport governing bodies. However, such proposals in the past have met opposition, although more authorities are now becoming convinced that this is the only effective way to stop the use of these drugs. An agreement was reached at the beginning of 1989 between the U.S. Olympic Committee and its counterpart in the Soviet Union to begin year-round testing of each other's international-caliber athletes. This was followed at the end of 1989 by a similar multinational agreement involving eleven countries: Australia, Bulgaria, Czechoslovakia, Federal Republic of Germany, Great Britain, Italy, Norway, South Korea, Soviet Union, Sweden, and the United States. This program, supervised by the IOC Medical Commission, involves testing anytime throughout the year. Athletes are given up to forty-eight hours' notice to report to a testing laboratory in their own country. The testing procedure is observed by representatives from at least one of the other countries involved in the agreement. Interest has been expressed by several other countries, such as Canada and the German Democratic Republic, to join in this agreement. This may prove to be a major step forward in the battle to control drug use in international sports.

A program of random, year-round testing for anabolic steroids was part of the drug-testing proposal developed for the NCAA by its original panel of experts in 1984, but this part of the proposal was quickly dropped by athletic administrators before it could even be considered by the NCAA membership. More recently, the NCAA has begun a year-round testing program for anabolic steroids, but it is a *voluntary* program. At the time of this writing, a plan was being developed for consideration by the NCAA membership to institute year-round *mandatory* testing for anabolic steroids. The recommendation is that for the first two years of the program, testing be done only for Division I football, only for anabolic steroids, diuretics, and other urine manipulators, and that a school be given forty-eight hours' advance notice of testing. After two years on this limited trial program, testing could then be expanded to other sports. The NCAA finally appears to be recognizing the futility of testing for this class of drugs only at championship events. Despite a few highly publicized positive tests for anabolic steroids during the first couple of years (e.g., Brian Boswell of the University of Oklahoma), very few positive tests for anabolic steroids have been detected at championships and football bowl games.

It might be argued that this means the tests are working in that they are deterring anabolic steroid use, and therefore the number of positives should be expected to be low. Based on experience in international sports, this is highly unlikely. The international experience has clearly shown that the only practical way that use of anabolic steroids will be deterred throughout the year is to make the athlete susceptible to testing throughout the year. However, any attempts by sport governing bodies in this country to test year-round for anabolic steroids may run into problems because of the "fall-out" from the legal controversies over the NCAA's decision to test for street drugs as well as performance-enhancing drugs and their apparent failure, as outlined in the previous section, to maintain a clear distinction between these two types of testing.

CURRENT STATUS OF DRUG TESTING IN U.S. SPORTS

Level of Drug Use Among Athletes

While there are many studies of street-drug use among people of various age groups in the general population, there have been very few studies of drug use among athletes as a special group. Most of the studies done on athletes have been done at one or two schools, which do not necessarily make the results generalizable to all athletes. The public perception of a major street-drug problem in athletics is based on media coverage and other anecdotal reports. The few studies that have been done have consistently shown that street-drug use by athletes is no greater than that of the general population of the same age, and for some drugs it may even be less.

Only two national-scale studies have been done on drug use patterns of athletes, the first in 1984 by the Office of Medical Education Research and Development at Michigan State University (Anderson & McKeag, 1985) and the second was a replication of the first study, done in 1988, by the same group (Anderson & McKeag, 1989). These studies were done on national samples of male and female college athletes in a variety of sports and were funded by the NCAA. They are the only studies currently available that can reasonably be generalized to a national population of athletes, in this case to college athletes. The results of both studies indicated that, as with the earlier small-scale studies, street-drug and alcohol use was no greater, and in some cases less, than for the general population of that age group (see Table 6.2). By far the most commonly used drug is alcohol.

TABLE 6.2 Drug Use in a National Sample of College Athletes[a]

Type of Drug	Percentage Used in Past 12 Months	
	1984	1988
Alcohol	88%	89%
Marijuana/hashish	36	28
Major pain medications	28	34
Cocaine/crack	17	5
Amphetamines	8	3
Anabolic steroids	4	5
Psychedelics	4	4
Barbiturates/tranquilizers	2	2

Source: Adapted from Anderson & McKeag (1985) and Anderson & McKeag (1989).
[a]1984 Total = 2,039 (male = 1,407; female = 632).
 1988 Total = 2,282 (male = 1,552; female = 730).

Both the 1984 study and the 1988 replication cited above found that a majority of the athletes supported some form of drug testing of athletes. Another interesting finding from the first study was that, for all but one street drug, most athletes who had used a particular street drug had begun use while in high school or junior high school rather than after they had begun college. The exception was cocaine, where half of those who had used it had done so in high school or junior high school, and half after beginning college. Four years later, the 1988 study showed that cocaine is now most often first used prior to entering college, as was indicated by 69 percent of those who had used cocaine.

The 1988 replication study showed that over the four-year period since the initial study there was a moderate decrease in the percentage of college athletes using marijuana, a moderate increase in use of major pain medications, a significant decrease in the percentage using cocaine and amphetamines, and a moderate rise in the use of anabolic steroids (Table 6.2). The percentage of athletes using anabolic steroids varied considerably by sport. While all five men's sports surveyed (football, basketball, track and field, baseball, tennis) contributed to the overall 5 percent usage rate, the greatest use was in football, with 10 percent of the players saying they had used anabolic steroids in the previous twelve months, and track and field, with 4 percent. In 1984 only one (swimming) of the five women's sports surveyed (swimming, basketball, track and field, softball, tennis) showed any usage of anabolic steroids; in 1988 three of the five women's sports (basketball, swimming, track and field) showed 1 or 2 percent of their athletes using anabolic steroids. The 4 to 5 percent usage rate for anabolic steroids found in these studies is considerably less than the general public perception of the level of use based on media reports. But it is still much greater than the percentages of athletes who test positive in the NCAA testing at championships and bowl games, which is less than 1 percent each year. This tends to confirm that testing only at these events does little to discourage use of this type of drug and does a poor job of catching those who do use anabolic steroids.

While there now is a small amount of data on college athletes, there are no similar data available on street-drug use patterns of professional athletes. Professional teams apparently have been somewhat reluctant to cooperate with such studies. At the moment, the only information we have is the growing number of media reports of professional athletes being suspended or being sent to treatment programs, which seems to indicate a relatively high proportion of this small, select population has developed a drug problem. However, as was illustrated by the difference between perceptions based on media reports and actuality based on research data for college athletes, this is not a solid basis for drawing conclusions. Several people involved with professional sports have claimed that the athlete's drug problems do not begin after they reach the professional level, but are picked up and brought with them from college. But the data on college athletes shows no more than the usual amount of street-drug use among college athletes, and most who do use drugs began in high school or ear-lier. Obviously, it would be helpful to have more dependable data on drug-use patterns in professional athletes.

Drug Testing in Professional Sports

Despite strong objections to drug testing from some professional athletes and their unions, some drug testing does take place in professional sports, although it generally is limited compared with that seen in amateur sports. What follows are brief summaries of the status of drug testing in various professional sports.

Football

National Football League (NFL) players are tested at preseason camps, and only for "reasonable cause" during the remainder of the season. Non-playing NFL employees may also be tested. Players testing positive may receive outpatient counseling and a thirty-day probation, or thirty-day inpatient treatment; after three positive tests, the player is banned from the NFL. Testing is done for amphetamines and other stimulants, street drugs (e.g., cocaine, marijuana), and anabolic steroids. Although for sev-eral years the NFL has had a policy against the use of anabolic steroids, until now there has not appeared to be as much interest in enforcing this policy as there has been in responding to the public concern about street drugs. While there are numerous reports of players testing positive and being treated for use of street drugs, similar reports of players using an-abolic steroids are conspicuously absent despite the statements of several players that use of anabolic steroids is not uncommon in the professional ranks. The NFL's image in this regard was not helped when at least one NFL team contacted Canadian sprinter Ben Johnson about a tryout for the team within a few hours after the gold medal he had won in the 100 meter dash at the 1988 Olympic Games in Seoul had been taken back because of a positive drug test for anabolic steroids.

Basketball

The National Basketball Association (NBA) has had a collective bargain-ing agreement with the players' association ever since 1983 that limits testing only to cases of "reasonable cause." If a player with a drug prob-lem voluntarily seeks help from the league, he receives his salary and free treatment. The second time this occurs, the player again receives free treatment, but loses his salary. The third time, the player is suspended for life but may petition for reinstatement after two years. If a player does not voluntarily seek help, but tests positive, he is permanently suspended. The only drugs for which the players are tested are cocaine and heroin. A recent agreement between the NBA and the players' association al-lowed random testing of all first-year players in NBA training camps, starting with the 1988–89 season. If a new player tests positive, he is suspended and receives treatment. Once this same player tests negative, he is then subject to the regular drug-testing policy.

Baseball

Major League Baseball cannot test ballplayers unless they have a drug-testing clause in their contract or unless they have known involvement with drugs. In an apparent effort to put pressure on a reluctant players' association, the commissioner of baseball instituted a random testing program for all others involved with Major League Baseball, including owners, executives, managers, and umpires. The drugs tested for include cocaine, marijuana, heroin, and morphine. There is no specific set of penalties for a positive test; each case is handled individually by the commissioner's office.

Boxing

The World Boxing Council (WBC) requires testing of both participants in any WBC world title fight. The testing takes place immediately after the fight, and is done for a list of drugs similar to the IOC list. Any boxer who tests positive is suspended for two years from any WBC-recognized fight and loses any WBC title he may hold. The World Boxing Association (WBA) has no drug-testing requirements for WBA-sanctioned fights, and in the United States it is left to each state to control.

Tennis

The Men's International Professional Tennis Council (MIPTC) tests at no more than two MIPTC tournaments each year. Testing begins on the first day of the tournament for players, staff, officials, and committee members, and continues until all have been tested. The drugs for which testing is done are cocaine, heroin, and amphetamines. Players who test positive must undergo treatment. Three positive tests for an individual, or failure to enter a treatment program after testing positive, results in suspension with reinstatement considered after one year. The U.S. Tennis Association adheres to the same policy for its professional members, while following the United States Olympic Committee (USOC) policy for its junior level (amateur) players.

Hockey

The National Hockey League does not have a drug-testing policy.

Soccer

The Major Indoor Soccer League has no drug-testing policy.

Drug Testing in College Sports

Both the history and the development of the NCAA drug-testing program have been outlined earlier in this chapter. Ever since the 1986 fall season, the NCAA has been testing athletes at NCAA championships in selected sports and postseason football bowl games, which are the only events over which the NCAA as an organization has direct control. In individual sports the top-place winners and other randomly selected participants are tested; in team sports the participants to be tested are selected on the basis of position or playing time, with other randomly selected team members also tested. Testing is done for the IOC drug list plus street drugs, although the NCAA has eliminated corticosteroids, narcotic analgesics, and sympathomimetic amines from its list. At this time the testing of the urine samples, which are collected and transported according to essentially the same strict chain-of-control standards as developed by the IOC, is done only at the three IOC-certified laboratories in North America (Los Angeles, Montreal, and Indianapolis). The development of a certification program to identify a number of regional labs throughout the United States that could be used by the NCAA and its membership is being discussed. The NCAA also has developed a voluntary program of testing, primarily for anabolic steroids, that can take place anytime during the school year, although there is a possibility that this program will be replaced by a mandatory year-round testing program.

Any athlete testing positive under the NCAA program is declared ineligible for postseason championships or football bowl games for a minimum of ninety days. If the athlete tests positive a second time, postseason eligibility is lost for two seasons. In individual sports (e.g., track and field, swimming, wrestling), any place finishes and team points won by an individual are vacated and team scores adjusted accordingly to determine team championships. In team sports (e.g., football, basketball, ice hockey), the situation is a little more complicated. There have been some very lively discussions within the NCAA membership regarding whether or not an entire team should be penalized if one of its players tests positive. For instance, should a basketball team that has won its first two games in the NCAA postseason tournament be declared ineligible if the test result from the first game for one of its players comes back positive? What if that player did not play in the first game? What about the teams that lost to this team? And, of course, what about the money the school is to receive for taking part in the tournament, which increases with each succeeding round of the tournament? A number of ways of handling this problem have been proposed. Initially, the entire team was penalized if one player who participated in a game tested positive, but that was quickly changed to declaring only the individual player ineligible, as a temporary way to handle the problem until a consensus of the membership can be reached.

Another problem that caused a modification of the original penalties for a positive test was the issue of an "indirect" positive test for marijuana. The testing methods are sensitive enough that it was felt that an athlete might test positive for marijuana even if he or she was not smoking it, but was in a closed room or car where it was being smoked by others. To compensate for such a possibility, the first positive test for marijuana results in a warning; a second positive test results in loss of eligibility.

Over the past few years an increasing number of colleges and universities have implemented drug-testing programs for athletes, usually in conjunction with or as a part of drug-education programs. As already mentioned, virtually all of these testing programs are for street drugs, with the accompanying legal complications discussed earlier. Very few test for the primary performance-enhancing drugs, namely anabolic steroids. However, testing for anabolic steroids is a very complicated and very expensive process, and few schools can afford to do any extensive testing for these drugs. Many schools have been using inexpensive field test kits to test their athletes. While these kits are less expensive, they also are less accurate than laboratory testing with gas chromatography and mass spectroscopy. The field test kits also are useless for testing for anabolic steroids.

A number of the smaller colleges and universities belong to another collegiate sports-governing body, the National Association of Intercollegiate Athletics (NAIA). These institutions are generally equivalent to the Division II and Division III schools of the NCAA. After some early experimentation with drug testing at a few national championship events in 1985, the NAIA has chosen not to involve itself in drug testing, primarily because of the expense for its smaller schools with smaller athletic budgets. However, the NAIA required that all of its members have a drug-education policy or plan in effect by the end of 1988. Each member school must submit a review of the operation of its drug-education program to the NAIA national office on a yearly basis. A few individual schools do test their athletes for street drugs, but generally not for anabolic steroids because of the expense.

Drug Testing in High School Sports

The national governing body for high school sports is the National Federation of State High School Associations (NFSHSA). Unlike the NCAA and NAIA, which enforce a set of regulations and procedures for member schools, the NFSHSA is primarily a service organization, providing rule books for various sports and suggested policies that the state high school associations may or may not adopt. The primary authority for governing high school sports lies within each of the state associations. The NFSHSA, therefore, as an organization has not been promoting drug testing at the high school level, but since 1985 has been developing and promoting a model drug-education program for use by the state associations and individual high schools. A small number of high schools around the country have implemented drug-testing programs for athletes, testing for street drugs, but because of legal concerns, these testing programs in most cases are voluntary.

Drug Testing in National- and International-Level Amateur Sports

The basic elements of drug testing in amateur sports outside the high school and collegiate setting have been presented earlier in this chapter, in relation to the IOC and USOC drug-testing programs. At the international level the IOC is the leading organization, monitoring the recent multinational year-round testing agreement and setting the standards for testing at the Olympic Games. These standards generally are followed by other international sport governing bodies at major international competitions. The penalties by the IOC for testing positive at the Olympic Games include banishment from any further competition in the current games, loss of any medals won and any records set, and any other penalties that might be imposed by the international sport governing body involved and the national Olympic Committee of the athlete's own country. Penalties by international sport governing bodies vary from sport to sport, but most commonly include exclusion from any competition sanctioned by the international body for a period of two years. Reinstatement is possible after the two years, possibly sooner upon petition by the athlete. Recently there has been discussion within many of the international governing bodies about making the penalties more severe. There also have been major meetings to discuss standardizing testing procedures and penalties across all sports.

Within the United States the situation is similar to the international picture. Ever since the 1983 Pan American Games, the USOC has had an ongoing drug-testing and education program, based on the IOC program, and now is part of the multinational year-round testing program monitored by the IOC Medical Commission. The USOC tests at the annual Olympic Festivals in the years when the Olympic Games are not held, and it oversees testing at the national trials for the teams to be sent to the Olympic Games, the Pan American Games, and the World University Games. Many national governing bodies for each sport test at national championship events, often with the support of the USOC. The drugs tested are from the IOC list of performance-enhancing substances, and the penalties for a positive test generally are similar to those of their respective international sport bodies.

FUTURE DEVELOPMENTS

As mentioned earlier, there is a continuous "race" between athletes who feel they have to use drugs and therefore look for ways to circumvent drug tests and those who are responsible for doing the testing and therefore must keep up with or keep ahead of the ploys engineered by the athletes. Just as a major war forces rapid developments in medicine and

certain types of technology, this "war" between drug users and drug testers will result in rapid development of testing methodologies and experimentation in new ways to artificially enhance athletic performance.

Some of the recent methods used by athletes are causing concern.
Some athletes have reportedly begun trying human growth hormone
(HGH), instead of anabolic steroids, to get the effects of the steroids without the danger of being detected. This is because currently no test exists
to detect HGH use. One of the side effects from the use of HGH is acromegaly—overgrowth of bones in the hands, feet, forehead, nose, and
jaw. Until recently, HGH was very scarce, the only source being the pituitary glands of cadavers, with many pituitary glands being needed to
produce a small amount of HGH. However, advances made over the past
few years in genetic engineering have made possible the development of
bacteria that can produce large amounts of HGH. Even though HGH is
not currently detectable, athletes apparently have not been rushing to use
this suddenly more readily available drug because of the adverse side effects. Research to develop a test for externally administered HGH is
being done.

Another performance-enhancing technique that has become more
prominent in recent years is blood doping, or the removal and freezing of
approximately a pint of blood from an athlete several weeks before a competition, and then reinfusing it into the bloodstream just prior to the competition. During the weeks after withdrawal of the athlete's blood, the
body produces new red blood cells to replace those withdrawn. The rein-
fusion of the additional red blood cells has the effect of increasing the
oxygen-carrying capacity of the blood, which can be critical in endurance
sports such as distance running, distance swimming, cycling, or cross-
country skiing. The resulting increase in aerobic capacity may be relatively small, meaning a few seconds improvement, but even a small increase can spell the difference between a first-place finish and finishing
back in the pack in competition at the international level. When done
properly, there apparently is little health risk in blood doping, other than
the normal risks of infection when transfusing blood, when using the athlete's own blood. However, blood doping becomes a much riskier procedure when another person's blood is transfused into the athlete, as was
done to several members of the U.S. cycling team during the 1984 Olympic Games. The risks include transmission of blood-borne diseases (e.g.,
hepatitis, AIDS) and adverse reactions of the body to incompatible components of nonhomologous blood.

Presently, there is no test available to detect blood doping in an athlete,
although a possible testing procedure is being developed and evaluated in
Europe. Normally the IOC does not ban a performance-enhancing drug
or technique unless there is a test available to detect it. In this case, however, the IOC (and the USOC) in 1986 formally banned the use of blood
doping to enhance athletic performance. Blood doping has pushed the
limits of the usual distinction between ethically and philosophically ac-

ceptable and unacceptable means of enhancing athletic performance (e.g., weightlifting vs. drugs). The usual definition of "unacceptable means" has centered on use of any substance foreign to the body with the sole intention of increasing athletic performance in an artificial manner. The athlete's own blood definitely is not a foreign substance, so the definition now includes any physiological substance taken in abnormal quantity or taken by an abnormal route of entry into the body. It is presumed that testing technology will soon catch up with the practice of blood doping.

A very recent development that will push the ethical and philosophical limits even further is the potential availability of erythropoietin (EPO). This is an experimental drug for treatment of anemia that acts to stimulate red blood cell production in the body. In essence, this drug has the potential to provide the same effects in an athlete as blood doping, without the risks involved in transfusing blood. EPO apparently disappears from the body in a matter of a few days, leaving an increased red blood cell count. Currently there is no test for EPO, but the drug also is very difficult to obtain since it is still experimental. However, when EPO becomes more generally available through the use of genetic engineering of bacteria, it will pose a problem for athletic officials, on both technical and philosophical grounds.

Major developments in drug testing of athletes in the near future likely will come in the courtroom. The greatest volume of activity is, and will continue to be, at the collegiate level. Most of the schools that will respond immediately to public concern about drug use in sports by developing testing programs have probably already done so. Others are no doubt waiting for the legal dust to settle before making any decisions on implementing a drug-testing program. Meanwhile, the number of drug-education programs will continue to increase. Legal challenges will likely eliminate a number of the more poorly designed testing programs (and perhaps even a few well-designed ones). Groups such as the NCAA and the American Council on Education have been developing guidelines and model testing programs to help schools avoid some of the legal pitfalls, as they are known at the moment. In general, they recommend that (1) drug-testing programs must have a specific, well-defined purpose; (2) a clear written policy must be provided to all athletes outlining the testing program and the consequences of a positive test; (3) informed consent should be obtained from each athlete; (4) confidentiality should be maintained; (5) the testing procedures should be of proven accuracy; and (6) due-process procedures should be adhered to throughout the program.

Beyond these general guidelines, it is difficult to provide a single good model program because situations vary greatly from one institution to another. As an example, some schools may have to deal with more complex legal concerns than others, because some constitutional provisions apply differently to public schools compared to private schools, and local statutes may have a major impact on a drug-testing program. For instance, the state Constitutions of California and Washington have more explicit provisions concerning right to privacy than does the U.S. Constitution. It is apparent that the results of the numerous legal challenges will be the major factor shaping the future of drug testing in American sports during the years ahead.

SUMMARY AND CONCLUSIONS

Two major themes appear to have been developing in the United States in recent years with regard to drug testing in sports; these themes center on the media and the courts. The first concern has been the impact of the print and electronic media on the growth of drug testing in athletics in this country. As a result of being placed in the limelight by the media, the problems of the athletes as well as their accomplishments receive inordinate attention. When the problem of alcohol and particularly street-drug use became a major focus of media attention in the early 1980s, the resulting public pressures led to a major increase in the number of drug-testing programs, primarily at the collegiate sports level. These same public pressures and concerns, shaped by the media's focus on street-drug problems in society in general and professional sports in particular, led colleges and universities to direct their drug-testing efforts primarily at street drugs rather than the well-established historical concern of drug testing in sports, namely the performance-enhancing drugs.

As a result, the second theme recently has come to the fore, which is the impact of the courts on drug testing of athletes, as embodied in the many legal challenges currently making their way through the legal system. In response to public concerns resulting from media coverage of the drug-related problems of professional athletes, the decision by the NCAA and its member schools to include street drugs in their drug-testing programs has resulted in a number of court challenges. Most of these challenges would likely have been on less solid legal ground, or never have been made, had the drug-testing programs followed the well-established precedent of testing only for drugs that enhance athletic performance. Because the clear distinctions between testing for performance-enhancing drugs and testing for street drugs have not been maintained by the collegiate community, there exists a potentially serious threat to the ability of non-collegiate sports authorities, such as the USOC, to test for performance-enhancing substances should the courts make sweeping decisions against the collegiate testing programs. Failure to maintain the distinctions between the two types of drug testing does not allow the courts to address the legal concerns that are primarily related to street-drug testing, while leaving undisturbed the established principles of testing for performance-enhancing drugs. While there undoubtedly will be new advances over the next few years in the laboratories with regard to performance-enhancing technology, and matching advances in testing technology, the most important aspects of the future of drug testing in sports in this country will be shaped in the courtrooms.

As long as drug testing in sports retains its historic, narrowly defined focus on ensuring fair competition by testing only for performance-enhancing drugs, it remains on solid philosophical and legal ground that has been accepted by society and the courts over the years. However, when athletic drug testing ventures into the area of testing athletes for so-called recreational or pleasure-enhancing drugs, it becomes a highly questionable enterprise subject to the same philosophical and legal challenges that are quite appropriately facing drug testing in the workplace and other areas of society. Whether or not the rationale of the athletic establishment for instituting testing of athletes for pleasure-enhancing substances (i.e., for the "health and safety of the athlete," which is a separate issue from "ensuring fair competition") is of overriding importance is a highly debatable issue at this time. However, the athletic establishment should realize that, in pursuing this course, it runs the very real risk of losing in the courts its well-established right to test athletes for performance-enhancing drugs as long as it fails to make a clear distinction between testing athletes for pleasure-enhancing drugs and testing for performance-enhancing drugs.

REFERENCES

Anderson, W.A., & McKeag, D.B. (1985). *The substance use and abuse habits of college student athletes.* Research Papers No. 1 and No. 2. Available from the Office of Medical Education Research and Development, East Fee Hall, Michigan State University, East Lansing, MI 48824.

Anderson, W.A., & McKeag, D.B. (1989). *Replication of the national study of the substance use and abuse habits of college student athletes.* Available from the Office of Medical Education Research and Development, East Fee Hall, Michigan State University, East Lansing, MI 48824.

Catlin, D.H. (1987). *Detection of drug use by athletes.* In R.H. Strauss (Ed.), *Drugs and performance in sports.* Philadelphia: W.B. Saunders.

Fraleigh, W.P. (1985). Performance-enhancing drugs in sport: The ethical issue. *Journal of Sport Philosophy, 11,*23–29.

Murray, T.H. (1983, August). The coercive power of drugs in sports. *The Hastings Center Report,* (Briarcliff Manor, NY), pp. 24–30.

Murray, T.H. (1986). Drug testing and moral responsibility. *Physician Sportsmedicine, 14*(11),47–48.

Reese, D., & Underwood, J. (1982, June 14). I'm not worth a damn. *Sports Illustrated,* pp. 66–82.

7

Drug Testing in Private Industry

HELEN AXEL

Ever since the early 1980s, drug testing has gained increasing acceptance among major U.S. corporations as a workplace strategy for controlling substance abuse. Surveys conducted within the past year, including one from The Conference Board in 1988,[1] estimate that approximately half of the nation's largest firms are testing both applicants and/or employees for drug use. Current estimates reflect substantial growth in the number of drug-testing programs since the early and mid-1980s.[2] Results of The Conference Board's survey, reviewed in this chapter, provide an overview of drug-testing experiences in large corporations.

The proliferation of drug-testing programs has not occurred without controversy and legal challenge, however, and testing remains limited in scope and largely confined to the job applicant population. New insights from The Conference Board's survey reveal that most employers proceed cautiously when investigating and implementing drug-testing programs. It is apparent among these major corporations that drug testing is not considered or used as a stand-alone "quick fix," but rather as one component of a comprehensive corporate policy constructed to deal with a serious and complex workplace problem—a multifaceted strategy that also includes employee counseling and assistance services, drug education, and training for employees and supervisors, and, to a lesser extent, special security measures.

SCOPE OF THE CONFERENCE BOARD SURVEY

A clear majority of the 681 companies responding to The Conference Board's survey (hereafter the Board) reported they tested applicants or active employees for drug use, or were in the process of implementing a drug-testing program. The survey was conducted by mail among 2,675 of the largest corporations in manufacturing; gas and electric utilities; finance and insurance; transportation; wholesale and retail trade; and other—primarily service—industries.[3] On average, returns from manufac-

140

TABLE 7.1   Respondents and Response Rates of Drug Testing by Industry

Characteristic	Number	Rate (%)
Total sample	681	25.5
Manufacturing	262	26.5
Finance, insurance	186	25.8
Utilities	104	38.8
Other industries	129	18.6

Note: Although these survey responses appear low, they are considered above average in research involving employers. An acceptable overall response rate in surveys of corporate executives conducted by The Conference Board is 20 percent.

turing firms and financial institutions were close to, but slightly above, the overall response rate of 25.5 percent, while participation among the utilities was significantly higher, and responses from the other industry groups surveyed were well below the average (see Table 7.1).

Manufacturing and financial businesses together comprised two-thirds of the respondents, utilities accounted for approximately 15 percent, and transportation, trade, and other industries constituted the remainder. Somewhat more than a fourth of the firms surveyed employ fewer than 1,500 workers in the United States, but 44 percent have more than 5,000, and 13 percent reported at least 25,000 employees.

EXTENT OF DRUG TESTING

According to the Board's survey, the incidence of drug testing is highest among manufacturing, public utilities, and transportation firms, and lowest in the financial-service sector (see Table 7.2). Consistent with this industry pattern, it is not surprising that companies with drug-testing programs tend to have male-intensive work forces. They also have a high proportion of skilled craft and production workers and a strong union presence.

Size of firm is also a factor: Companies with 10,000 or more employees are more than two and one-half times as likely to test applicants and/or employees for drugs as are those companies with fewer than 1,500 workers. To a certain extent, size of firm in this study can be explained by industry composition. For example, about half of the companies with work forces of fewer than 1,500 were banks, insurance companies, and other financial institutions—an industry sector in which only 13 percent of the firms overall are engaged in drug testing. On the other hand, 54 percent of the corporations with 25,000 or more employees are in the manufacturing sector, where 64 percent of the firms have drug-testing programs. Still, some differences may, in fact, be attributable to size alone. For example, smaller manufactures and utilities—industries where drug-testing programs are generally widely accepted and used—are also

TABLE 7.2   Prevalence of Drug Testing

Characteristic	Percentage of Firms with Drug-Testing Programs
Total sample	49%
Industry	
Manufacturing	64
Finance, insurance	13
Utilities	79
Other industries	49
Domestic work force	
Under 1,500	29
1,500 to 5,000	44
5,000 to 10,000	48
10,000 to 25,000	69
25,000 and over	81
Headquarters location	
Northeast	48
North-Central	49
South	58
West	41

less likely to do drug testing than are the larger employers within these sectors.

Regional variations in the extent of drug testing can also be partially explained by industry and size differences among the survey participants. However, even when industry and size characteristics are accounted for, drug-testing programs are more frequently employed in the South and Middle Atlantic states than they are by firms in New England and on the West Coast. The low-incidence regions include states in which laws protecting employee rights are particularly strict. Although the geographic analysis is based on the address of the corporation's headquarters rather than a distribution of its employee population, a sizable proportion of the company's work force is likely to be located in the region of the corporate address. In addition, because policies are normally determined at the corporate level, local employment conditions will undoubtedly have some influence on the policy developed.

Drug testing is essentially a U.S.-based program. Although half of the survey participants are multinational firms, very few have any substance-abuse programs that extend beyond national borders.

CLIMATE FOR DRUG TESTING

How do employers perceive substance-abuse problems at the workplace and what particular conditions contribute to their decision to develop drug-testing programs? It seems clear from the Board's survey that business executives who hold different views about the severity of drug problems are certain to have different attitudes and responses toward drug testing. It is also clear that the nature, size, and location of the business also help shape the company's response.

Perceptions of Substance-Abuse Problems and Trends in Use

Over three-fifths of the companies that are currently testing for drug use during the employment process—or among groups in their active employee population—perceive substance abuse to be a multidimensional issue in which both alcohol and illegal drugs are involved. By contrast, a similar percentage of employers not engaged in drug testing regard alcohol as the major drug of abuse in their work forces. Financial institutions and smaller firms are most likely to view substance abuse in this light. But a near majority of all the firms surveyed concur that chemical dependency affects employees in all types of jobs and at all levels in the organization. They also are in agreement that certain geographic sites seem to be more susceptible than others to substance-abuse problems.

Comparing the present with the recent past, nearly half of the officials from firms in the drug-testing group believe that problems with illegal drugs have grown worse, adding such comments as "cocaine and crack are more readily available," "marijuana has become more acceptable," "more hard drugs are evident," and "we have more polydrug users now." Executives in the utilities and transportation industries appear more pessimistic about the spread of drug use than are officials in other firms. But several company executives dispute this assessment, maintaining that management's greater awareness of drug use, not an actual increase in the problem, is really the most significant development in the last few years.

Although about a third of the managers in the nontesting group of companies acknowledged concern about growth in employee use of illegal drugs, three out of five found no increase in drug problems or claimed ignorance regarding recent trends. "We do not see drug abuse as a serious problem," "we have only had one alcohol abuser in the past five years," "we don't have specifics, but substance abuse is not a problem in our employee group" are some of the comments included on their surveys. Because many of the respondents in this group are executives in smaller firms, the likelihood of more direct contact with their employees may lead them to believe they have a better grasp of the situation—or perhaps make them unwilling to admit that individuals known to them can have drug problems.

Initiatives to Combat Substance Abuse

The Conference Board survey found, in general, that companies engaged in testing for drug use are consistently more active on a number of fronts in their battle against workplace substance abuse than are their nontesting counterparts. To be specific, these firms are far more likely to have formal substance-abuse policies, coordinated efforts toward drug education, and employee assistance and counseling programs (EAPs). And these programs usually exist in combination with each other: In a typical firm engaged in drug testing, the company will also have a written policy, an EAP, *and* an active drug-education program in place. Special security measures, though not widely used, are still more likely to be present when drug testing is conducted.

However, as previously described, drug-testing firms have distinct industry and size characteristics that contribute to these differences. For example, larger corporations tend to develop "program" responses to their workplace problems more often than smaller firms, where ad hoc approaches and informal arrangements are prevalent. In addition, some industries, particularly in the manufacturing sector, have long track records in dealing with addictive disorders at the workplace, a situation that may make them receptive to new initiatives in this problem area. Thus, while a number of comparisons are drawn between drug testing and nontesting firms in this review, the reasons for their differences may lie elsewhere.

Formal Substance Abuse Policies

For most corporations, a written substance-abuse policy is a prerequisite for drug testing: Policies are present in nine out of ten companies that are screening applicants or employees for drug use.[4] A substantial majority are of recent origin, 1986 or later, or were updated since 1985. At minimum, virtually all current policies cover employee use of both alcohol and illegal drugs. In addition, more than six companies in ten also encompass prescription medicines and other mind- and behavior-altering substances, and over a fourth are directed at employee behavior both on and off the job.

According to the survey, a cross section of disciplines within drug-testing firms have participated typically in the policy development. Most frequently involved are representatives from the human resources, legal, security, medical, and labor relations units and, to a lesser extent because they are not universally present, the employee assistance program. Just a fifth of the firms with unionized work forces included union representation in the discussions. Although sometimes not a direct participant in the policy development process, the CEO almost always is closely identified with the final document and its official promulgator.

Just as many points of view are solicited in developing a substance-abuse policy, so too companies with drug-testing programs use many channels of communication to make sure that employees and supervisors understand the conditions of the policy—and the penalties for failure to abide by them. Both verbal and written communications are involved. For example, detailed procedures are available to supervisors in over 80 per-

cent of the corporations surveyed. And three-fourths of the firms discuss
the company's position on alcohol and drug use during orientation programs for new hires, as well as in training sessions for current employees
and managers. Employee handbooks, articles in company publications,
videos, and posters provide additional vehicles for publicizing company
standards and expectations about substance-abuse issues.

Substance-abuse policies are present in somewhat more than half of the
firms participating in the Board's survey that do not test for drug use. But
fewer viewpoints are incorporated in their design, and detailed guidelines
are more often than not unavailable to supervisors. Moreover, these employers tend to rely primarily on written documents—such as employee
handbooks—to notify employees about company policies. Orientation
and training sessions, staff meetings, and other forms of face-to-face ex-
changes are far less common.

Drug Education and Awareness Programs

In addition to communicating company policies, a significant majority of
the corporations surveyed are engaged in some form of drug education,
including direct preparation of special materials or programs and the distribution of information developed by noncorporate sources. As with
substance-abuse policies, however, larger firms, particularly those with
drug-testing programs, are most likely to have developed or sponsored
educational materials about drug use and abuse.

Although corporate educational initiatives appear extensive among the
corporations surveyed, the target audiences are largely confined to the
firm's immediate constituency—its employees. Dependents are half as
likely to be the beneficiaries of these efforts, and less than one company
in ten reported distributing materials to school children, community res-
idents, or other segments of the general population.

Employee Assistance Programs

A key component of many corporate substance-abuse initiatives is the
employee assistance or counseling service program (EAP). Early EAPs
evolved from occupational alcoholism programs that were prominent in
the manufacturing industries from the World War II era until about 1970.
During the 1970s, the EAP movement experienced a big surge in growth
when "broad brush" counseling services for family and personal problems were added to the core EAP mandates. But stepped-up drug trafficking activity and the increased availability and use of illegal drugs during this decade have provided even greater momentum to the spread of
EAPs, just as other substance-abuse control measures have also become
more prevalent.

As evidenced in the Board's survey, the 1980s have been a very active
period in the EAP movement throughout the corporate community. Seven
out of ten companies studied started their employee assistance programs
during this period, and more than half implemented EAPs within five

years of the survey date. Drug-testing firms are more likely to have somewhat longer experience with their EAPs, but many appear to have launched them in very recent years, along with a number of other measures to deal with workplace drug problems. In aggregate, employee assistance programs remain more evident today in firms where drug testing is also present—76 percent of these companies have EAPs, compared with 58 percent in the nontesting group.

The recent increase in corporate-sponsored employee assistance programs appears to have been facilitated by rapid growth in the number of national and local contractors for EAP services. Outside providers, which administer over half of the employee assistance programs identified in The Conference Board's survey, are used by more than 60 percent of the companies that do not have drug-testing programs. Forty-five percent of the drug-testing firms, on the other hand, have an in-house capability for providing assessments and, sometimes, limited counseling and treatment to employees seeking the service. EAPs in these firms also seem to handle more problems related to substance abuse, although these statistics are difficult to interpret since drug and non-drug problems are often interrelated. No significant distinctions are apparent between companies with and without testing programs in the availability of EAP services: Employees and their dependents in all or most locations generally have access to them.

Special Security Measures

Media reports of draconian security measures used in some firms to eliminate drug trafficking, possession, and use have brought cries of alarm about a growing "police-state mentality" at the workplace. But these concerns appear to be inconsistent with reality, according to survey findings. Locker, desk, and vehicle searches, gate checks, drug-sniffing dogs, and similar measures are infrequently used by employers expressly for drug-control purposes. And although special security procedures are more prevalent in companies that have drug-testing programs, even in this group only about a third of them engage in such activities. As a rule, most of the action on the security front (with regard to drugs) has taken place in the last five years, and most procedures are in effect at a restricted number of sites. Security measures to control drug use are virtually nonexistent in companies without drug-testing programs.

REACHING A DECISION TO TEST FOR DRUGS

Based on findings from the Board's survey, drug testing is a strategy not lightly undertaken. Many players are involved in researching the issue, and the investigation usually takes months—sometimes years—before either a positive *or* negative decision is reached. Although there is some indication that firms seriously considering, but ultimately rejecting, the concept of drug testing conclude their investigations more quickly than do companies that adopt testing programs, only a fourth of all employers in the Board's survey required less than six months to make up their minds. In a third of the firms, at least a year elapsed before a decision was made.

Conditions Influencing the Decision

Many of the same departments that contributed to the firm's new or revised policy on substance abuse are involved in the drug-testing decision. However, because drug testing is generally regarded as a policy issue and medical matter, security department views are sought less frequently when such programs are under review. The employee assistance unit has been a contributor in more than a third of the discussions that have led to drug-testing programs.

Company officials cite evidence of drug problems in the workplace as the single most compelling reason for considering—and implementing—a drug-testing program. As earlier data have shown, corporations with drug-testing programs appear more acutely aware of substance-abuse issues and more decisive in their actions. A greater sensitivity toward—and willingness to acknowledge—drug-abuse problems among their employees has undoubtedly made these firms more receptive not only to drug testing but also to a variety of other substance-abuse control measures.

The belief that testing for drugs can assist managers in the early detection of drug use before addictive behavior takes hold, and before drug problems become more serious at the worksite, also leads employers to explore a testing strategy. In the view of many proponents, drug testing not only has the capacity for detecting incipient drug problems but can also act as a deterrent to others who may be tempted to experiment with drugs. In addition, using drug testing as an employment screening procedure, many proponents argue, sends an important signal into the community that the company will not tolerate drugs at the workplace and that drug users will not be hired. Because many employers recognize that community drug problems can become workplace problems, pre-employment screening is frequently intended as a preventative measure. When other employers in the area test job applicants, such procedures become even more appealing. No company wants to be seen as a haven for drug users.

Legal considerations also rank high in the decision process. Many corporations say they have initiated testing procedures to detect applicant or employee drug use—or are now leaning toward such a strategy—because they are worried about their legal liability in the event of drug-related accidents or incidents. Some employers already have faced costly legal battles, while others anticipate them because of the types of jobs their workers perform. Publicity surrounding drug incidents in such industries as nuclear power plants, airlines and trucking firms, and a variety of manufacturing settings—to say nothing of the growing drug-crime link—has certainly raised the public's awareness of the potential for danger when drugs are present.

In addition to high visibility in the media, businesses also pay attention to statistics on the high cost of workplace drug use—including data on lost time, accidents, drug treatment and related health care expenses, employee theft, and the like. Available national estimates can be persuasive, and a few employers also have gathered compelling statistics about conditions in their own companies.

In various combinations, the factors outlined here may contribute to a company's decision to launch a drug-testing program. They also undoubtedly are responsible for other company initiatives in the war against drugs. But some other considerations were found to be distinctly less important. For example, about two-thirds of the employers surveyed said neither consultants' recommendations nor negative publicity about company-related drug problems factored into their drug-testing decisions. In addition, a significant majority of the respondents denied being swayed by success stories about government/military testing programs.

Companies That Said No to Testing

Some firms eventually decide that drug testing is not an appropriate "solution" for them. At the time they were surveyed, 8 percent of the corporations without testing programs indicated that they were proceeding to implement such a program, while another 7 percent said they would start an investigation in the near future. Most of the companies, however, had considered and rejected the concept of drug testing or expressed no interest in exploring its feasibility. (A sizable number of nontesting firms also chose not to answer the question.)

When asked what reasons employers had for their decision not to test, the ones most frequently mentioned are the threat of legal action challenging the testing procedures or issues involving the employer-employee relationship. Other major reservations concern the accuracy of the tests, testing's inability to measure impairment, the potentially negative impact on employee relations, and perceived incompatibility with the firm's philosophy. The issue of corporate culture is a particular stumbling block for the financial services industry, where respondents also tend to minimize the extent of drug use in their work forces, even dismissing drug testing as unwarranted.

CHARACTERISTICS OF
DRUG-TESTING PROGRAMS

Who is tested and under what circumstances, how the program will be managed, how the testing will be conducted, and what actions will be taken against individuals who test positive for drugs are all questions that need to be addressed before an effective drug-testing program can be mounted. Many details about the testing procedures, not reviewed in this summary, also need close examination so as to assure integrity of the collected specimens and validity of the testing process. Although differences exist in details, many similarities are apparent in the core elements of the testing programs examined.

When Testing Is Done and Who Is Tested

Pre-employment and for-cause testing are the two most prominent types of drug-testing programs in use today, based on results of the Board's survey. More than nine out of ten companies that have a drug-testing program screen applicants, and somewhat more than seven in ten report that accidents or incidents, suspicious behavior, and other conditions specified by the company's policy trigger drug tests for active employees. Altogether, however, less than fifth of the firms have totally "externalized" their drug-testing activity by confining the procedure to the employment process.

Three-fourths of the companies conduct pre-employment screening and testing for cause in combination with one other form of drug testing—usually as a means of monitoring employees who are or have been in treatment for drug use. Testing for drugs during routine physicals or other periodic exams is far less common, and only thirty companies in the Board's survey population reported they had random-testing programs. Applicant testing is also present in virtually all of the firms with periodic and random-testing programs.

Very few of the companies studied have extensive experience with drug-testing activity. Just 10 percent of the 845 individual types of programs acknowledged by the survey respondents were initiated prior to 1983, but well over two-fifths date from 1987 and early 1988 (when the survey was in the field). *All* of the random-testing programs identified were implemented in the post-1983 period. Because a number of plans were reported to be in the works at the time of the survey, and another group of companies indicated they were about to launch investigations, the proportion of companies inexperienced in drug testing is likely to remain high over the next few years.

Of all the forms of drug testing, pre-employment screening is the most "universal" program, usually affecting all persons seeking employment at all company locations—although firms generally restrict test procedures to serious candidates or finalists for available positions. In most corporations, too, for-cause testing and testing for monitoring purposes are applicable to all employees under conditions outlined in the company's policy. Periodic and random testing, however, more typically affect only certain job categories (including, for example, individuals who operate heavy equipment or have other jobs that present danger to themselves or others), or certain job sites.

In aggregate, then, relatively few employees appear to be directly affected by the proliferation of drug-testing programs. Much of the testing activity today is in the applicant population, and defined circumstances almost always limit its use among active employees. A Department of Labor survey issued in early 1989 confirms this assessment. Results from the government study show that less than 1 percent of employees in private nonfarm business establishments were tested for drug use between mid-1987 and mid-1988, although about 20 percent of the employees were in worksites where testing was done.[5] Studies of government testing programs also reveal that few employees in the public sector have been exposed to these procedures.[6]

Program Management and Administration

Management patterns for drug-testing programs reflect the corporation's organizational structure and reporting relationships. For the most part, drug testing is a headquarters-driven program. The corporate staff is responsible for developing the policy, and administrative authority for the testing program remains at the corporate level. Top management is directly linked through the chain of command to the program's operation.

In well over half of the companies, the drug-testing policy and procedures are uniform throughout the organization and the program is administered by headquarters staff. In another third, individual business units within the firm maintain operational control over testing procedures, but a corporate manager coordinates these activities and reports to top management.

Major elements in the drug-testing process appear quite uniform from company to company, a consistency that probably can be attributed to the acceptance of basic industry standards by major drug-testing laboratories, the principal providers of drug-testing services to these large employers.[7] In addition, two-thirds of the survey respondents contract with only one testing laboratory, and three-fourths engage the outside laboratory to perform either all sample collection and testing procedures or all testing of samples collected on-site by company medical personnel.

Company officials note that uniformity in the testing process is critically important, and restriction in the number of laboratories and personnel involved is one way to minimize deviations. However, about a fifth of the employers surveyed acknowledged that local variations occur in the testing procedures, which, some of these respondents admit, interfere with the successful operation of the program.

Consistency is apparent elsewhere, too. The widely recommended assays for broad screening purposes—TLC (thin-layer chromatography) and immunoassays (such as the EMIT, produced by Syva Company, and the Abuscreen, from Roche Diagnostics)—and gas chromatography/mass spectrometry (GC/MS) for confirmatory tests, are used by nine out of ten firms in the survey. The overwhelming number of employers test for recent use of a variety of drugs including, most commonly, cocaine and its derivatives, marijuana and other cannabinoids, opiates, barbiturates, and amphetamines. Benzodiazepines and PCP (phencyclidine) are somewhat less frequently found on the list of drugs to be identified. About half of survey respondents test for alcohol use, though rarely with breathalyzers. One company in four uses some other biological samples (such as blood, saliva, or hair) in their screening processes.

Consequences of Positive Test Results

Job applicants who test positive for drug use can almost always expect to be denied employment. In seven out of ten firms, this decision is based on confirmation of the preliminary screen. A somewhat larger majority of companies accept reapplications from candidates who have been rejected for drug use, but keep their test records on file and require a waiting period of at least several months before new applications can be submitted. One-fourth of the employers, however, refuse to reconsider the candidate for any future position once drug use has been detected.

When active employees are subjected to drug tests, confirmation tests are more common, but still not universal. Virtually all employees with test-confirmed drug problems have access to the employee assistance program and, in fact, are strongly urged to seek help. As a rule, job applicants cannot avail themselves of the company's EAP services, although a handful of companies report such opportunities are provided.

Clear-cut mandates for particular courses of action against employees who have tested positive for drug use are rare. Most company policies are written to allow for discretion and consideration of extenuating circumstances in individual cases. However, the survey results show that, on average, employees are more likely to be *disciplined* following first confirmation of drug use and can expect to be *discharged* on a second positive drug test. Action dictated by lack of cooperation from employees who undergo counseling and treatment is less clear, although failure to complete a prescribed treatment regimen and refusal to submit to drug tests for monitoring purposes after treatment appear to be grounds for termination more often than not.

LEGAL CHALLENGES AFFECTING EMPLOYERS

Twelve percent of the companies conducting drug tests among applicants and/or employees reported they had been challenged in the courts because of their testing program. Twenty-three percent said they had been involved in arbitration cases. Although some experience with multiple arbitration cases was evident in this small group of employers, most companies indicated they had dealt with only one or two cases, either in the courts or before arbitration judges. The newness of most drug-testing programs in the survey population, and their focus on applicant testing, may help explain why relatively few firms have faced legal confrontations to date.

Despite the limited number of corporations involved, conflicts between drug testing and employee rights have become high visibility issues in the press. Over half of the cases in litigation that were identified by the survey respondents, and about a third of those in arbitration, have centered on the testing process itself—the accuracy of the test results, and the procedures used to assure sample integrity and validity of the tests. Cases involving invasion of privacy have also been raised in courts and at arbitration hearings. Union representatives in arbitration proceedings have focused on wrongful discharge, violation of work rules, and failure of the employer to bargain as the bases for their complaints. In the experience of the companies surveyed, relatively few cases have involved complaints of intentional infliction of emotional distress, defamation, or handicap discrimination.

THE CORPORATE EXPERIENCE:
MANAGERS' PERSPECTIVES

Although few have hard evidence to back up their claims, corporate executives appear generally satisfied with their drug-testing experiences.[8] They are particularly emphatic about the testing program's positive effect on the quality of job applicants and the safety of the work environment. Even so, a substantial number of employers express less certainty about other benefits of drug testing. Two-fifths, for example, admitted they had no information about what effect drug testing has had on reducing drug-abuse problems in the workplace, and nearly half of the respondents did not know how job performance had been affected, if at all. A very small number of employers thought their drug-testing programs had depressed employee morale and weakened the credibility of the EAP, but these opinions were far outweighed by positive views.

A larger group of corporate executives, however, conceded that their drug-testing programs had encountered some difficulties. At the top of the list, as evident from previous observations, were employee resentment and/or union opposition. More than a fifth of the respondents found such resistance in their work forces. A similar percentage observed that conflicting interpretations of company policy were sometimes present, while somewhat smaller numbers were concerned about cheating in the sample-collection process, and uncertainties created by the evolving case law in the drug-testing process.

Summing up, executives who participated in the Board's survey are in accord with regard to recommendations to other companies contemplating drug testing. Most important, they stress that drug testing is not a cure-all—or a substitute for good management practice. They emphasize that companies should do thorough research, proceed slowly, and implement a comprehensive substance-abuse program. Corporations should also keep in mind, they say, that a clearly written corporate policy, extensive and continuous employee education and supervisory training, and a well-funded, supportive employee assistance program, all operating in concert with drug testing, may be the most effective strategy for controlling substance abuse in the workplace. Although remaining vigilant, a majority of these employers are optimistic. They believe, as one corporate medical director observed, "It is possible to manage drugs at the workplace and do it well."

NOTES

1. This chapter is adapted from Helen Axel, *Corporate Experiences with Drug Testing Programs,* Report No. 941, New York: The Conference Board, 1990.

2. See, for example, surveys conducted by the Employment Management Association (1986), the American Society of Personnel Administrators (1986), the College Placement Council (1986), Business and Legal Reports (1987), and the American Management Association (1987). A discussion of these and several other studies can be found in Thomas E. Backer, *Strategic Planning for Workplace Drug Abuse Programs* (DHHS Publication No. ADM 87–1538), Washington, DC: Alcohol, Drug Abuse and Mental Health Administration, U. S. Department of Health and Human Services, 1987, pp. 22–23; and *Employee Drug Testing: Information of Private-Sector Programs,* Washington, DC: United States General Accounting Office, March 1988. Comparative results from earlier surveys by some of the organizations are also provided. More recent surveys, indicating a continued trend, have been issued by the Bureau of National Affairs Personnel Policies Forum (1988), the Gallup Organization for Hoffmann-LaRoche (1988), and William M. Mercer, Inc., for Marsh & McLennan Companies (1988).

3. For additional details concerning The Conference Board's survey methodology, see Helen Axel, "Characteristics of Firms with Drug-Testing Programs," in Steven W. Gust and J. Michael Walsh, eds., *Drugs in the Workplace: Research and Evaluation Data,* National Institute on Drug Abuse, Research Monograph Series No. 91 (DHHS Publication No. ADM 89–1612), Rockville, MD: U.S. Department of Health and Human Services, Alcohol, Drug Abuse and Mental Health Administration, 1989.

4. The Drug-Free Workplace Act of 1988, signed into law by President Ronald Reagan on November 18, 1988, can increase the prevalence of workplace programs to control the sale and use of illegal drugs. The law requires federal contractors to provide workplaces that are free of illegal drugs. Among the specific requirements are a published policy statement, and a drug-free awareness program about the dangers of drug use and the availability of employee counseling, assistance, and rehabilitation programs. The law became effective March 18, 1989.

5. The government's analysis is based on business "establishments"—that is, individual plants, stores, or other work sites—rather than companies. Although conceptually different from The Conference Board's survey in this respect, the Department of Labor study is consistent with its findings when very small establishments are excluded. The nationwide probability sample survey, conducted

among 7,502 establishments, is the first survey on drug testing to encompass all sizes of establishments in all private nonagricultural industries. The establishment sample includes single-site small businesses, the majority of which are not engaged in any drug-testing activity.

6. The pool of government employees in sensitive jobs who are eligible for random drug testing is about one in twenty. Michael Isikoff, "Many are Called But Few Are Using Drugs," *The Washington Post National Weekly Edition,* July 25–31, 1988.

7. Mandatory guidelines for drug-testing programs in the federal work force, issued April 11, 1988, set certification standards for laboratories involved in urine testing for federal agencies. These standards provide a basis for evaluating the qualifications of testing labs used in the private sector. A list of federally certified labs has been published by the National Institute on Drug Abuse. In addition, some states regulate drug-testing laboratories. See *Employee Drug Testing: Regulation of Drug Testing Laboratories,* Washington, DC: United States General Accounting Office, September 1988.

8. Few companies have attempted to analyze the effects of their drug-testing programs, although aggregate data and trends in test results are tracked over time. Among the companies surveyed, only 10 percent had conducted evaluations of their programs—most frequently though internal records on absenteeism, turnover, accidents, employee theft, and similar data. For a compendium of workplace research on the impact of drug use and drug-testing programs, see National Institute on Drug Abuse [citation in note 3].

8

Substance-Abuse Testing in the Workplace: Legal Issues and Corporate Responses

ROBERT T. ANGAROLA

DRUG TESTING: RECENT EVENTS AND RESPONSES

Drug abuse in America is a problem everyone today recognizes. Employers are now facing the challenge of how to deal with this unfortunate fact of life while protecting the rights of workers and the public.* Recently, many companies have instituted comprehensive drug-abuse prevention programs aimed at improving employee health, safety, and productivity. Most of these programs have some form of drug testing as one element.

The issue of drug testing in the workplace has spawned literally hundreds of issues and sub-issues. Like the Greek Hydra, no sooner is one concern addressed than others spring up. This pattern of growth shows no signs of slowing down. The past three years have seen a rapid growth in the number of employers using urinalysis to test employees for substance abuse. Suits brought by employees and unions have risen proportionately.

Events in the past year shifted the focus of the drug-testing debate. The highly publicized overdose deaths of college basketball star Len Bias and pro football player Don Rogers brought the drug crisis to the front pages of every newspaper and centered attention on the use of testing as a preventative and rehabilitative tool in reducing drug abuse. In September 1986, President Ronald Reagan issued an Executive Order seeking a "drug-free Federal workplace."[1] The order declared that "[p]ersons who use illegal drugs are not suitable for Federal employment" and ordered agency heads to "establish a program to test for the use of illegal drugs

*Courts and legislatures continue to address the issue of substance-abuse testing. Their actions can affect employers' and employees' rights in this area. Companies should always consult with local counsel on any decisions relating to current or planned workplace substance-abuse programs that include testing.

155

by employees in sensitive positions."[2] The sixteen fatalities resulting from the January 1987 crash between an Amtrak passenger train and a Conrail freight train dramatized the tragic consequences of drug use by workers.

A recent California survey revealed that 85 percent of the respondents said that airline pilots, police officers, firefighters, and truck and bus operators should be required to submit to mandatory drug testing. Seventy-seven percent said that they would be willing to submit to random testing for drugs. Of those surveyed, drug use was considered the most important problem facing their community.[3]

Clearly, most Americans are willing to consider the use of drug testing in the workplace, for at least some jobs, as a necessary step to help ensure safety and productivity. The military and most large corporations in the United States are now using some form of drug testing. The debate is no longer *whether* any drug tests should be conducted, but rather *how* and *on whom* these tests should be performed.

Drug Testing: Responses in the Public and Private Sectors

This chapter discusses the legal issues involved in setting up and maintaining a comprehensive drug-abuse prevention program that includes testing for drugs. Several recent court decisions relating to government workers have provided many commonsense considerations that private employers should keep in mind when setting up a testing program. Employers are wisely erring on the side of caution in designing drug-abuse prevention programs that include drug testing.

In 1982, fewer than 5 percent of the Fortune 500 companies were testing employees for drug use. Today, almost half of those firms are conducting these tests in one form or another, and more are expected to follow. Among the companies that are reported to be using urinalysis to test all job applicants for drug use are IBM, Exxon, DuPont, Lockheed, Federal Express, Shearson Lehman, Hoffmann-La Roche, The New York Times Co., United Airlines, Boeing, and Trans World Airlines. Companies reported to be testing not only applicants but also certain current employees include Rockwell, Southern Pacific, and Georgia Power.[4]

Drug testing of government employees continues to increase. The military has been using drug testing for many years, and the services have been joined by such federal agencies as the Postal Service, the FBI, and the Federal Railroad Administration. In the near future the Drug Enforcement Administration (DEA) will start random drug testing. Local firefighters, police officers, and operators of buses, trains, and subways are being tested. Prison facilities all over the country are testing both correctional officers and inmates. A Virginia county operating the nation's largest school bus fleet has proposed a drug-testing program for its drivers.

To reduce drug abuse in the workplace, companies and government agencies are taking action to improve the health of their workers, protect the safety of the public and other employees, and preserve and improve the quality of their products and services.[5] They are not setting up "gotcha" programs aimed at prying into their employees' personal lives and firing drug users. Economic factors (theft, workplace accidents, absenteeism, higher health care costs) are a major consideration in setting up a drug-testing program, but there are also less tangible reasons. Companies whose employees abuse drugs suffer a negative public image, have low employee morale, lose the public's trust, etc.

Most of the companies that have set up testing programs provide their employees with opportunities to seek counseling or treatment for their drug problems and these services almost always are provided at company expense. These employers recognize that their workers are their most important assets. They also realize that drug testing alone is not sufficient to deal with the problem. Further, they know that workers must have access to employee assistance programs and other services that can keep them on the job and help build a healthier and more productive work force.

Yet there are frequent media reports of workers claiming that drug tests are an unwarranted and "unconstitutional" intrusion into their private lives. Generally, the courts have disagreed and sided with employers on the constitutionality of drug testing. This is because the parties claiming that drug testing encroaches upon the boundaries of their constitutional rights to privacy, fairness or due process are reflecting more their individual attitudes than an understanding of the law. Companies and, in most instances, employees recognize that comprehensive programs dealing with drug abuse improve health and safety in the workplace in a manner that is reasonable and effective. For example, the Southern Pacific Railroad reported a 71 percent reduction in accidents and injuries attributed to human error after it began its drug and alcohol program.[6] The Georgia Power Company stated that the accident rate at its Vogtle nuclear power project has decreased steadily since its comprehensive drug program was set up, from 5.4 for every 20,000 manhours in 1981 to 0.49 in 1985, a 90 percent decrease.[7] The military has reported a drop in drug use from 48 percent in 1982 to under 3 percent today. While officials state that this is "largely due to the drug testing,"[8] it is important to note that, in addition to a testing component, all these programs include drug-education activities and access to treatment services for workers who require them. These marked reductions in prevalence of substance abuse demonstrate another benefit of comprehensive abuse programs: their deterrence value.

Developing a Comprehensive Program

Urine testing for drugs is an important and useful tool. However, it can be effective only when it is part of a comprehensive program that addresses the health, safety, and productivity concerns of both the employer and the employee.

All successful drug-abuse prevention programs include certain key elements:

- Documentation of both the *need* for drug testing and the resulting *benefits* once testing is instituted.
- Education of employees on the health and safety implications of drug abuse as well as the employer's policies on employees who abuse drugs or alcohol.
- Training of supervisors to recognize substance abuse and to guide the employee into drug counseling and treatment programs.
- Rehabilitation and counseling opportunities for employees shown to be using drugs.

This chapter discusses the kinds of legal challenges being brought against employers using drug testing to detect substance abuse. It also suggests ways for private employers to defend legal challenges to their drug-testing programs or, better yet, to avoid them altogether.

While most of the cases discussed concern testing for drugs, the issues they address go beyond the tests themselves into all aspects of an employee substance-abuse program. Any company with a drug abuse prevention program—and that should be every company—needs to follow the principles that these cases stand for in identifying and dealing with employees with drug or alcohol problems.

CONSTITUTIONAL RESTRAINTS ON GOVERNMENT EMPLOYERS

The courts, while generally upholding most forms of drug testing, are developing an emerging set of rules as to when testing is appropriate and how such testing should be conducted to protect the rights of employees. The following sections discuss applicable legal principles, court-defined parameters, and commonsense rules that can help in developing a successful drug-abuse prevention program.

Note that the law is evolving rapidly in this area and that state and local statutes can affect what employers may or may not do. Companies should consult with legal counsel (as well as other concerned individuals) before instituting a substance-abuse program that involves drug testing. This is particularly true if there is going to be random testing of current employees.

The clash between changing social attitudes and the law as it affects employee drug testing has led to several legal attacks on the program. These challenges have centered in five areas: the right to privacy, the right to be free from unreasonable searches, the right to due process, negligence law, and labor law. In addition, workers have claimed that testing is a violation of federal or state rehabilitation acts that protect handicapped individuals. What follows is a discussion of each of these areas.

Right to Privacy

Americans hold two contrasting notions of the "right to privacy." The first is the common notion defined by each individual's personal belief of which aspects of his or her life are private and, being private, are not subject to intrusion by others. Social attitudes are reflected in how we draw the lines around our private lives. When we think these lines are crossed, there will be an outcry: "It's not the business of my boss what I do on Saturday night!"

The second notion is the constitutional "right to privacy"; this is the right to privacy that is legally enforceable and which protects far fewer activities than the average person's notion of privacy rights.

While some state constitutions contain such clauses, there is no specific provision in the U.S. Constitution guaranteeing a right to privacy.[9] The United States Supreme Court has held, however, that such a right is implied by reading several constitutional provisions together.[10] This constitutional right to privacy has been held to protect individual decisions on matters such as marriage, family, and childbearing. While the use of marijuana, cocaine, and other abusable drugs unfortunately has become commonplace—and even socially accepted in some circles—it never has been held to come within that zone of activities protected by the constitutional right to privacy.[11] Moreover, this constitutional right to privacy protects people only against *governmental* intrusion. Individuals acting as private citizens and private employers are not bound by these constitutional restraints.[12] However, private employers should develop drug-testing programs that comply not only with a legally enforceable right to privacy but also a reasonable worker's notion of a right to privacy.

Freedom from Unreasonable Searches
Judicial Opinions

While the term "right to privacy" often appears in media reports of challenges to employee drug testing, the fact is that most court claims of an invasion of privacy have been based on the Fourth Amendment prohibition against unreasonable searches and seizures by government authorities.[13] Plaintiffs assert that urine testing intrudes so far into an employee's privacy that it constitutes an unreasonable search in violation of the Fourth Amendment. Workers raise this argument not only against government employers, but also against private employers. Once again, however, the constitutional protection against unreasonable searches protects only against unreasonable *governmental* interference. When a private business is testing its employees for drugs, there is no government involvement and therefore no violation of this constitutional guarantee against unreasonable searches.

Note, however, that courts may apply this standard to private employers when they are operating under a government contract or when they are part of a highly regulated industry. In these cases, private sector employees may also be allowed to assert the Fourth Amendment right against unreasonable search and seizure.

Public employees can claim this constitutional right. Nevertheless, several courts have found that even government employees, performing certain duties, have less of a right to expect privacy than do others and therefore cannot maintain that a drug test is an unreasonable search. For example, a recent federal district court case upheld the testing of Washington, D.C., police officers suspected of drug use.[14] The court reasoned that

> [w]hile as a matter of degree we do not necessarily extend to the uniformed civilian services the same narrowly circumscribed expectation of privacy accorded to members of the military, the fact remains the police force is a paramilitary organization dealing hourly with the general public in delicate and often dangerous situations. So we recognize that, as is expected and accepted in the military, police officers may in certain circumstances enjoy less constitutional protection than the ordinary citizen.[15]

Testing of other government workers has withstood recent challenges that it violates the Fourth Amendment. In a case decided in a federal court in Georgia, city employees working around high voltage electric wires argued that urine testing violated their Fourth Amendment rights.[16] The court agreed with the terminated employees that the testing was a search, but said that because "the government has the same right as any private employer to oversee its employees and investigate potential misconduct relevant to the employee's performance of his duties, . . . the employee cannot really claim a legitimate expectation of privacy from searches of that nature."[17] The court balanced the intrusion of an employment-context drug test against the employer's need to determine whether employees engaged in hazardous work are using drugs. It found that the Constitution was not violated, because the search was a *reasonable* one. A key element was the fact that this search was not intended to uncover criminal activity but to help ensure a safer workplace.

In March 1987 a federal district court in Alaska ruled that while urine testing for drugs of certain Federal Aviation Administration (FAA) employees was a Fourth Amendment search, "public safety considerations outweigh the intrusion upon petitioners' legitimate expectation of privacy."[18] In other words, this court determined that the testing of these employees for drugs of abuse was not unreasonable in light of their responsibilities in ensuring the safety of the traveling public.

Drug-testing programs involving public employees or employees in a highly regulated industry have been upheld as constitutional by all four federal appeals courts that have considered the issue. The earliest case involved a union challenge to the constitutionality of a drug-testing program for city bus drivers.[19] The program contained a reasonable suspicion requirement; that is, drivers were tested only if they were suspected of being under the influence of drugs or alcohol *or* if they were involved in a "serious" accident. A lower court had found that the testing program was constitutional and "both desirable and necessary" and "not . . . un-reasonable."[20] The U.S. Court of Appeals (Seventh Circuit), citing the strong public safety concerns, the "reasonable suspicion" requirement triggering the testing program, and the testing procedures, found that "[u]nder these conditions and because 'a valid public interest justifies the intrusion contemplated,' probable cause exists" and upheld the program.[21]

Ten years later a second federal appellate court upheld unannounced mandatory drug testing of jockeys, even in the absence of individualized suspicion that a jockey was using drugs or alcohol.[22] The court based its reasoning on the highly regulated nature of the horseracing industry (and corresponding diminished expectations of privacy) and the strong state interest in maintaining public confidence in the integrity of that industry.

The 1987 *McDonnell* vs. *Hunter* case concerning drug testing of prison employees bolstered the earlier *Shoemaker* decision involving jockeys.[23] In *McDonnell*, the court found that drug testing is a reasonable search, even absent individualized suspicion, for prison employees with daily, regular contact with prisoners in medium and maximum security prisons. The court pointed out that prison employees already have "diminished" privacy interests due to the need to maintain prison security. These interests are lessened further by the limited intrusiveness of the drug-testing program (the court held that random urinalysis testing was the "least intrusive" method of detecting drug use) and the absence of more effective means to control illicit drug use in the prison system.[24]

Finally, the constitutionality of the drug-testing program of the U.S. Customs Service was upheld in April 1987.[25] This case represented a union challenge to the Customs Service program requiring employees transferring to "sensitive" jobs to submit to urine testing for drugs. The court reaffirmed what most other courts have held—that urinalysis drug testing is a "search" under the Fourth Amendment. It found, however, that the search was reasonable and therefore constitutional where the government interest in public safety outweighed the social interest in privacy, where the test is of limited intrusiveness, and where the purpose of the test is administrative and not criminal.[26]

On the other hand, some courts have not permitted governmental testing programs to go forward. A federal district court in Tennessee held that the random testing of city fire fighters contemplated under the proposed procedures was unreasonable because the invasion of the individual outweighed the articulated need to search.[27] The court stated that the proposed testing of its fire fighters was "not justified at its inception" because the city did not have reasonable grounds for suspecting that the test would find evidence of illicit drug use.[28] Additionally, the court ruled that the scope of the search was not reasonably related to the circumstances justifying the search. The proposed testing was not limited to those fire fighters for which the city had reasonable cause to suspect illicit drug use, and it did not appear that the city expended any effort to use less intrusive methods to detect drug abuse such as personnel procedures to document symptoms of drug abuse (e.g., absenteeism, aberrant conduct, and financial difficulties).[29]

More recently, a state court in New Jersey invalidated a City of Newark directive that all members of the city police force's narcotic bureau have semiannual urinalysis drug testing, holding that it violated the *state* constitution's prohibition against unreasonable search and seizure, which the state court recognized may afford greater protection than that required under the Fourth Amendment of the U.S. Constitution.[30] The state court reasoned that this particular governmental drug testing of public employees was unreasonable because the city did not have probable cause to believe that drug use within the narcotics bureau was extensive, a reasonable suspicion that certain individuals were using illicit drugs, and any evidence that the public was endangered by drug use by police officers.[31] This decision highlights the importance of remaining sensitive to state constitutional and statutory issues and developments.

Because the Fourth Amendment does not constrain private employers, they have more freedom to conduct drug searches in an effort to detect and address substance abuse within a company. For example, when investigations linked several Burlington Northern Railroad train accidents to employee alcohol or drug abuse,[32] the railroad unilaterally implemented a surveillance and search program using dogs trained to detect drugs in order to stop on-the-job alcohol and drug use. The union protested that the dog surveillance program was an unconstitutional search. A federal court specifically held that the search was not unconstitutional since the railroad, a private entity, was not bound by the Fourth Amendment.[33] The court stated that there was "nothing prohibiting a private entity from requiring any person, including an employee, to submit to a 'search' . . . as a condition of entering that entity's premises, or refusing entry to any person believed to be in possession of an illicit substance."[34]

Arbitrators similarly recognize that the private employer's right to search is broad. A 1983 decision approved a company search of employees' lunch boxes, trousers, shoes, socks, lockers, and vehicles after reports that employees were bringing drugs and handguns onto company property.[35] The arbitrator explained:

> Arbitrators have consistently held that the employer has a right to conduct a search of lunch boxes, lockers and persons and that [penalties for] refusal to permit a search may include discharge. These arbitrators have been attentive to the motivation for the search and the circumstances under which it was conducted, attempting to balance the legitimate interest of the employer and the personal dignity of the employee.[36]

The arbitrator found that the search was motivated by the company's justifiable alarm at reports that employees were carrying drugs and handguns onto company premises. The company hired a professional security consultant, who conducted the search with as much regard for personal privacy as the legitimate ends of the search permitted. Although the timing of the search was unannounced, advance notice of the company's policy was posted on the company bulletin board, the production office, the change room, and the gates to the plant.

The arbitrator upheld this search because the employer was justifiably concerned about the health and safety of all his employees and conducted the search with reasonable regard to the personal privacy and dignity of the workers. The arbitrator also recognized that informing employees of the search immediately before it was conducted would destroy its effectiveness. He acknowledged, however, that the employer could accommodate both his own and his workers' needs by notifying them that he would conduct such searches in the future.

This case illustrates an important concept. Employers often can implement needed drug-abuse prevention, identification, and intervention programs without undue employee resistance if they clearly communicate what they intend to do, explain why a search program is necessary, and consistently enforce the policy that has been adopted.

Administrative versus Criminal Searches

Two recent opinions upholding the constitutionality of government drug-testing programs focus on the nature and purpose of the "search" involved in urine testing for drugs. In both cases, one involving the Federal Aviation Administration (FAA) and the other the U.S. Customs Service, the courts' rulings in part relied on the administrative nature of the drug-testing program.[37] In other words, the purpose of testing was rehabilitative rather than punitive and the drug test results were not used to bring criminal charges.

As a professor of administrative law has stated,

> when fire marshalls inspect a building, or safety inspectors examine a workplace, they usually do not act because they have probable cause to believe there is a specific violation. Rather, the principal justification for the search is to help obtain general compliance with the law by placing potential violators on notice that their transgressions will not go undetected. Uncovering specific violations is secondary in facilitative searches, and often leads to assistance in correcting problems rather than to punishment.[38]

The same author noted that "[t]he same may well prove to be true concerning drug testing since many argue that workers found to be using drugs should be provided help in quitting, and disciplined or dismissed only as a last resort."[39]

The courts in both the FAA and Customs Service cases found the respective programs to be administrative efforts aimed at improving employee and public health and safety. The careful design of the Customs Service drug program led the court to note that "the need for [Fourth Amendment] protection against governmental intrusion diminishes if the investigation is neither designed to enforce criminal laws nor likely to be used to bring criminal charges against the person investigated."[40] However, the need to test certain government employees or applicants must be demonstrated in conjunction with proof of the administrative function served by testing.[41]

Due Process

The Fifth and Fourteenth amendments of the U.S. Constitution require the government to provide a person with due process before depriving anyone "of life, liberty, or property."[42] This is a requirement that the government engage in a fair decision-making process before taking measures that affect an individual's basic rights.

The courts have held that the actions a government employer takes toward its employees must be reasonably related to their jobs. When the government plans to penalize employees, it generally must notify them in advance and provide them with an opportunity to defend themselves.

Due-process arguments made against government employers using drug testing generally claim that the tests are inaccurate, that the results are insufficiently related to work performance, or that the employee was punished as a result of a drug test without being afforded an adequate opportunity to contest the test results. Again, while private employers are *not* bound by the constitutional guarantee of due process, in the interest of fundamental fairness prudent employers allow workers an opportunity to discuss alleged drug use. Therefore, although the next few cases will deal again with government workers, they have relevance to private industry.

Accuracy and Reliability

Courts that have passed on government employees' challenges of urine testing have confirmed the accuracy and reliability of the tests. In a case decided in a Georgia federal court in 1984, municipal fire fighters and police officers argued that both urine testing and polygraph examinations were so unreliable that their use violated protected constitutional rights. The court examined the polygraph issue in detail and agreed that, in spite of the city's need to monitor police and fire services, the tests were impermissibly unreliable. The urinalysis challenge, however, was presented, discussed, and dismissed in a brief footnote, with the explanation that "the court is not persuaded that use of such testing procedures will violate plaintiffs' constitutional rights."[43] In an unrelated case, the Supreme Court of Georgia upheld a finding that drug-testing procedures were reliable when used as the basis for revoking parole.[44]

In the recent *von Raab* case, a federal workers' union unsuccessfully challenged the drug-testing program of the U.S. Customs Service.[45] The district court held that the testing was an unconstitutional violation of the

Fourth Amendment and, "because of its unreliability, the due process clause," even though this latter issue was not raised by the union.[46] The federal appeals court reversed, agreeing that the testing was a search under the Fourth Amendment but found it reasonable (and therefore constitutional) because of "the strong governmental interest in employing individuals for key positions in drug enforcement who themselves are not drug users and the limited intrusiveness of" the Customs Service program.[47] Concerning the due-process violation found by the lower court, the appellate court stated that "[t]he drug testing program is not so unreliable as to violate due process of law."[48] The court elaborated by pointing out the undisputed reliability of the gas chromatography/mass spectrometry (GC/MS) follow-up test and strict chain-of-custody procedures. Moreover, the Customs Service program would permit employees to resubmit samples reported as positive to a laboratory of their choosing. The court also looked favorably on the quality assurance features of the program (intermingling of control samples to track false-positive readings and regular quality assurance reports to the union).[49]

The Eighth Circuit Court of Appeals recently held that a positive enzyme-immunoassay test confirmed by a second such test contains sufficient indicia of reliability to provide some evidence of drug use that would allow prison officials to take disciplinary action against an inmate.[50] This case involved prisoners who, naturally, have a lessened expectation of privacy. Private and public employers always should use a radioimmunoassay or enzyme-immunoassay as a screening test and confirm positive test results with GC/MS or an equivalent process before denying a person a job or instituting disciplinary procedures.

Courts that have considered this issue have not found the lack of perfect accuracy in urine testing to be significant enough to serve as the basis for a successful constitutional challenge. Indeed, in an analogous situation, the U.S. Supreme Court has accepted the reliability and accuracy of breath-testing equipment.[51] The Supreme Court held in 1984 that due process did not require state police to retain the breath samples of suspected drunk drivers tested on a medical device called an Intoxilyzer. The Intoxilyzer measures the alcohol level of the breath of the person tested. Although, like urine testing, it may not be perfectly accurate, the High Court found that the possibility of a false positive (registering the presence of alcohol when none was there) was so slim that the preserved sample would have virtually no exculpatory value to the drunk-driving defendant. Therefore, the California police, though technically capable of preserving breath samples, were not required to do so because of the accuracy of the testing equipment.

"The materiality of breath samples," the Court reasoned, "is directly related to the reliability of the Intoxilyzer itself. . . . [I]f the Intoxilyzer were truly prone to erroneous readings, then Intoxilyzer results without more might be insufficient to establish guilt beyond a reasonable doubt."[52]

However, the justices believed that the testing device results were sufficient to establish guilt beyond a reasonable doubt because they found that the test was not prone to erroneous results.

The accuracy of the urine tests is close to 100 percent when, as recommended by manufacturers, positive results are confirmed by a second GC/MS test. As stated in a recent court decision involving the testing of flight service specialists, employees whose urine tests positive on an initial immunoassay test have their specimens retested using the highly accurate gas chromatography/mass spectrometer, which has been viewed by courts as "the most accurate test available."[53]

In contrast to breath-alcohol testing and urine testing, courts and legislatures have found polygraph examinations—lie detector tests—too unreliable to use even to support employment-related decisions. Recall the fire fighters' and police officers' challenge of lie detectors and urine tests. The court ruled that the city could not use lie detector tests to combat drug use among its police officers and firefighters, but it could use urine testing as the basis for disciplinary action. One-third of the states have laws prohibiting private employers from requiring employees to take lie detector tests.[54] Results of lie detector tests are generally inadmissible in court.[55] Arbitrators also refuse to consider results of lie detector tests as proof of the truth of the person's response.[56] However, this has not been the case with drug-testing equipment.

Relationship to Work Performance

The relationship between test results and work performance presents a more difficult legal question than does the accuracy of the test itself. At present, urine testing detects the presence of drugs or the metabolites of drugs in the body. Test results will be positive when an abusable substance or its metabolite is detected in the sample, even though the person tested may not presently be "impaired" or "intoxicated." Current technology cannot yet measure impairment.

Opponents of the test have argued that, since the mere presence of the tested substance does not necessarily mean impairment at the workplace or long-term intoxication, the results have no relation to on-the-job performance. However, longer-term impairment from the use of drugs is often difficult to measure. Reports of a recent Stanford University study of pilots who had smoked marijuana indicated erratic and potentially dangerous performance on a simulator twenty-four hours after use of the marijuana, long after any sensation of being high was gone.[57] In addition, theft and fraud in the workplace, drug dealing, absenteeism due to substance abuse, accidents, workers' compensation claims, increased health care costs, and decreased employee morale are connected with employees who use drugs on and off the job. Nevertheless, the relationship between test results and work performance at times presents difficult legal questions, both because of the intangible nature of adequate performance and the inability of the tests to measure impairment.

A Louisiana state court case involved a city van driver's disqualification for unemployment benefits because of misconduct on the job.[58] A coworker had admitted leaving the company building to smoke marijuana in the company van and was fired. The van driver, however, denied smoking marijuana on the job. When his urine test came up positive for marijuana, the city fired the driver for being under the influence of drugs during working hours. The driver had testified that while he had not smoked marijuana on the job, he had smoked it at 1:00 A.M. the day he was tested. He successfully argued at the administrative and trial court levels that the city had failed to prove that he was "intoxicated" on the job or that he was unable to perform his work in a safe manner because of his off-the-job behavior.

The state court of appeals reversed, ruling that it was an error to require the agency to prove intoxication or inability to work. "Merely smoking marijuana, or drinking alcohol or taking any other 'recreational' drug that may impair one's driving, while one is supposed to be working as a driver," the court explained, "is misconduct connected with the employment."[59]

The appellate court balanced the public interest against the employee's rights and found the test to present an acceptable answer to a serious employment issue. Nevertheless, the two lower tribunals did hold against the city. To avoid the problem of trying to link the presence of drugs to impairment, most companies adopt "drug-free" policies that make it a violation for employees to have illegal drugs or metabolites in their system on the assumption that the risks of drug abuse affecting performance negatively and causing safety hazards are reason enough to take disciplinary actions even without present intoxication.

Another aspect of this issue was discussed in a recently reported arbitration decision. The case involved a utility operator of paper machines who arrived at work in an unfit condition to perform her duties. Her employer requested that she submit to a drug test. The worker refused and she was fired. The arbitrator ordered the termination changed to disciplinary suspension with reinstatement but denied back pay and benefits. The arbitrator did not question the employer's right to request or require a drug test. However, in this instance the employee was requested, not ordered, to take such a test and the employer failed to advise her of the severe consequences of refusal.[60] This type of problem can be avoided by sound personnel policies and practices, as discussed in the next section.

Opportunity to Contest Results

The due-process guarantee of fair decision making also means that a government employer must provide employees with a reasonable opportunity to contest charges against them before they can be punished.

For example, a federal court has held that it is a violation of a government employee's right to due process of law to terminate that person's employment on the basis of a positive urine test without allowing the employee the opportunity to have an independent analysis of the sample.[61] Courts also have recognized the importance of an employee's right to a hearing on a decision to terminate employment based on a positive drug test, while finding that safety considerations may require holding that hearing after a person has been suspended from current duties.[62] The principle behind these decisions is that the "level" of due process afforded the government employee must be a reasonable one—reasonable based on all of the circumstances. These considerations of reasonableness, as well as a balancing of all relevant factors, should enter into any disciplinary decision based on drug testing. Private employers generally are not bound by the federal constitutional requirement of due process, but, as in other areas, reasonableness is the key when instituting any form of substance-abuse program.

Wise personnel practices, sound public relations, and most labor contracts require that an employee be given some notice of the reason for any disciplinary action and some opportunity to discuss that action with a superior. The private employer's best insurance against allegations of unfairness in disciplinary actions is to advise employees in advance what will happen should they test positive for drug use, refuse to take a test, or otherwise are identified as substance abusers. Supervisory personnel should offer to meet individually with employees to discuss work-related problems before discipline is instituted. (*Caution:* Supervisors should *not* discuss an individual's personal drug problems or accuse anyone of drug use—this should be handled by specially trained personnel.) Employers should consider retesting any worker who presents plausible objections to the results of a single positive urine test. Always err on the side of the employee.

LEGAL CONSIDERATIONS FOR ALL EMPLOYERS

Negligence Law

Unlike the constitutional claims just discussed, negligence claims can be brought against both private employers and government entities. Employee negligence actions against employers are generally of three types. First, an employer may be liable for negligence in hiring a substance abuser who harms another employee or the public. Second, an employer may be liable for negligence should the employer fail to conduct the drug-testing procedure with proper care. Third, while an employer has a qualified privilege to communicate test results to those in the company who need to know about them, an employer who maliciously spreads untrue reports of positive test results will not be protected from employees' charges of libel and slander.

Negligent Hiring

The importance of controlling substance abuse in the workplace assumes additional significance because of an employer's duty to foresee the dangers presented by an impaired employee or face substantial damages should the employer fail to do so. This principle is illustrated in a 1984 New Mexico case that involved a boy who was sexually assaulted by an intoxicated hotel employee. The employee had been fired from his job as a dishwasher because of drinking. The hotel later rehired him, even though other hotel employees knew that he regularly drank on the job. The boy's parents sued the hotel, claiming that the hotel was negligent in hiring and retaining the employee.

The appellate court found that there was enough evidence for a jury to decide whether the hotel should have foreseen, and therefore should be held responsible for, the employee's behavior. It sent the case back for a new trial so that a jury could decide on the hotel's liability and the amount of damages.[63]

This duty extends beyond visitors or guests of the company. All employers have an obligation to maintain a safe workplace for employees.[64] This obligation is not met when an employer hires an individual who injures co-workers as a result of a substance-abuse problem that an employer carelessly failed to detect.

The Occupational Safety and Health Act (OSHA) presents an additional reason for employers to be attentive to personnel hiring practices. The "general duty" clause of the act requires virtually all employers to provide

> a place of employment which [is] free from recognized hazards that are causing or are likely to cause death or serious physical harm to [its] employees.[65]

This clause taken alone does not justify drug testing of employees. However, because there have been reports that drug users have three times the number of accidents as nonusers,[66] this is a relevant fact for employers to consider. A recent Court of Appeals case in Washington, D.C., emphasizes this need. The court invoked the general-duty clause to impose liability on the employer, even though no specific regulations had been violated. The court stated that OSHA

> clearly and unambiguously imposes on an employer a general duty to provide for the safety of his employees that is distinct and separate from the employer's duty . . . to comply with administrative safety standards.[67]

Negligent hiring is an emerging area of tort law whose boundaries have yet to be defined. Most states, while recognizing it as a cause of action, prefer that plaintiffs first exhaust more traditional theories of recovery. Liability may be assessed where an employer knew or should have known that an employee "posed an unreasonable risk of harm."[68]

An established company policy and program against employee substance abuse, consistently enforced, could serve as an effective defense to a negligent hiring claim. An employer who has made clear that substance abuse on the job will not be tolerated, who has followed through with testing and other means of detection, who has offered rehabilitative assistance to substance abusers and, as necessary, has imposed sanctions will have a better chance of identifying and dealing with the impaired employee before he (or she) causes harm. Furthermore, the employer who has instituted and consistently enforced such a policy is also less likely to be held responsible for injuries caused by an employee who, without detection, violates the company's rules on substance abuse.

Negligent Testing

In 1982, two Michigan job applicants were refused employment after testing positive for drugs. They filed suit against the lab that performed the tests, and to buttress their claim that the lab was liable for negligent testing, they introduced into evidence the manufacturer's instructions that accompanied the testing apparatus, instructions that suggested that results should be confirmed by an alternate testing method. Because of its failure to follow the manufacturer's labeling, the laboratory agreed to a settlement with the two job applicants.[69] Similarly, the District of Columbia federal court has held that the firing of a school bus attendant on the basis of a single, unconfirmed positive urinalysis test was arbitrary and capricious. The local school board had announced in advance that *confirmed* findings would be grounds for termination. The court rejected as inadequate confirmation the school board's argument that it had repeated the test manually with the same test system that had been used before but with the addition of computer analysis, especially when the manufacturer's label on the test kit, a Food and Drug Administration report, and an advisory opinion from the Centers for Disease Control all indicated that positive results with this particular test system required confirmation by an *alternate* method.[70]

While negligent testing exposes an employer to greater risk, valid testing conversely helps insulate against successful lawsuits. Two applicants for fire-fighting positions sued the City of Detroit and the laboratory that had returned positive test results for marijuana. Based on these results, the city had revoked the applicants' certifications of eligibility for fire-fighting positions. The city had confirmed the test results as suggested by the manufacturer. A federal court dismissed the negligent testing claims even before the case reached trial.[71]

These cases show the importance of following manufacturers' instructions when conducting drug testing. But an employer's duty to test with care encompasses more than simply adhering to the instructions provided by the manufacturer of testing equipment. It also includes choosing a laboratory that ensures that personnel administering the tests are properly trained, that the tests will be performed fairly and accurately, and that adequate care will be taken to protect the chain of custody over the urine samples. Of particular importance, then, is selecting a lab with high quality-control standards and adherence to proper procedures. For example, some labs test several specimens with urinalysis drug-test reagents intended by the manufacturer for use on one specimen. If an employer is unwilling to absorb the cost of hiring a highly reputable laboratory, it should not institute a drug-testing program.

Libel and Slander

A bus driver for a major private transportation company was suspended from work after a drug test, which was given as part of the required company physical, was reported as positive for marijuana. News of his suspension and the test results spread to the bus driver's family, co-workers, and acquaintances. Two weeks after the first urinalysis, the bus driver was retested. The results were negative and the company reinstated him.

The driver sued the company and a state trial court awarded the driver $5,000 damages for libel and slander. The court held that the laboratory and the company physician, knowing the purpose of the test and the consequences of an erroneous report, showed reckless disregard for the truth by communicating the test results without ensuring that they were correct. The Tennessee Court of Appeals, however, reversed this decision, holding that there was no libel or slander because the plaintiff could not prove actual malice.[72]

On the other hand, in a Texas case, a railroad switchman sued his employer for libel and slander after urine test results falsely indicated the presence of methadone. The company physician who administered the urine test had explained to the company that further study would be required before he could draw any conclusions on drug use. Without any additional investigation, however, the company instituted disciplinary proceedings. A second urinalysis, performed at the employee's request, indicated that a compound was present in the urine sample that had characteristics of methadone but was not in fact methadone or any other commonly abused drug. The company nonetheless issued a statement that the switchman had been using methadone and that this justified his dismissal. This statement was circulated throughout the company and to outsiders. The switchman collected $150,000 for damage done to his reputation and an additional $50,000 in punitive damages from the railroad.[73]

These cases demonstrate that employers should confirm test results and should not publicize results beyond those individuals who absolutely need to know. As the Texas decision proves, errors in this area can cost many thousands of dollars.

Labor Law

An employer who plans to institute a drug-testing program or other means of detecting illegal drug use should determine whether the plan complies with employment or union contracts, and first renegotiate those contracts if it does not. In any event, management should inform the union of its intent to institute a drug-testing program and discuss the reasons for such a program with employee representatives.

Earlier, in the context of a private employer's right to conduct searches, this chapter discussed a union's lawsuit against the Burlington Northern Railroad. That case also raised a second issue of contract law when the union argued that the use of drug-detecting dogs, unilaterally implemented by the railroad, was in violation of the federal Railway Labor Act because it was a major change in employment conditions that was made without required union consultation. The railroad had a safety rule prohibiting on-the-job use or possession of drugs or alcohol; employees were well aware of that rule. The railroad argued that use of drug-detecting dogs in its search program was within its managerial discretion to enforce that no-alcohol, no-drugs rule. The court halted the program by agreeing with the union that the employer had changed the employment contract without the legally required union consultation. Even though there was already a rule banning drugs and alcohol on the job, a program to enforce that rule could be instituted only through collective bargaining between the railroad and the union.[74]

The language in an employment or union contract binds an employer and must be drafted carefully. One arbitrator held that a clause in a union contract prohibiting the "sale or use of intoxicants or drugs" did not prohibit a union member's *possession* of marijuana.[75] Obviously that employer did not condone workers bringing drugs onto the company premises as long as they did not sell or use them. The employer simply lacked the foresight to consider that the phrase he was using technically could be interpreted to exclude drug activity involving possession alone.

Labor arbitration cases often differ from court cases in this respect: the arbitrator's decisions may reflect conscious or unconscious bias in favor of allowing an employee to keep his or her job.[76] Companies therefore should be alert to the existence of any careless terminology in the employment contract that might permit an arbitrator to find a way to excuse instances of substance abuse.

Rehabilitation Act

The Drug Abuse Prevention, Treatment and Rehabilitation Act of 1972 prohibits denial of federal civilian employment, except for certain sensitive positions, to anyone on the basis of prior drug use, unless that person cannot properly function in his or her employment.[77] Similarly, the Rehabilitation Act of 1973 prohibits discrimination against any handicapped individual by any employer who receives federal financial assistance.[78] Some have argued that the federal Rehabilitation Act and similar state statutes prohibit the use of testing to identify employees or applicants who are using drugs. However, an analysis of the statute as interpreted by the courts indicates that the Rehabilitation Act probably will have little, if any, impact on the use of drug testing in the workplace.

It is clear that the Rehabilitation Act protects alcoholics and drug abusers from discrimination in employment.[79] The act prohibits such discrimination against former drug abusers as a group.[80] However, former drug abusers by definition should suffer no adverse effects from workplace drug testing since they are no longer using drugs.

The issue then becomes what effect the law may have on current drug users. While the Rehabilitation Act covers alcoholics and drug abusers, the protected class of "handicapped individual" is explicitly limited to exclude an

> alcoholic or drug abuser whose current use of alcohol or drugs prevents such individual from performing the duties of the job in question or whose employment, by reason of such current alcohol or drug abuse, would constitute a direct threat to the property or safety of others.[81]

Under this exclusion, all individuals who are impaired on the job and any drug user who holds a position that affects the safety of the public or other workers would not be considered "handicapped" and therefore would not be entitled to protection under the act.[82]

The only remaining group who might be affected adversely by workplace drug testing and arguably could be entitled to protection under the law are occasional or casual drug users. But, again, the definition of "handicapped individual," the prerequisite status for protection under the act, appears to exclude these people from coverage. The Rehabilitation Act defines a "handicapped individual" to be

> any person who (i) has a physical or mental impairment which substantially limits one or more of such person's major life activities, (ii) has a record of such impairment, or (iii) is regarded as having any impairment.[83]

Although work definitely is classified as a "major life activity,"[84] the courts have held that the ability to qualify for any one job or even a narrow category of jobs is not a "major life activity" if there are other options for satisfactory employment.[85] Therefore, occasional use of marijuana or other drugs, which would disqualify a person from certain jobs, such as police officer or fire fighter, would not necessarily be a "handicap" under the act.[86] Occasional drug use also would not constitute a physical or mental impairment that "substantially" limits a person's major life activities. The Rehabilitation Act appears to cover only the kind of chronic drug abuse that would prevent a person from performing substantially all jobs that might otherwise be available. In most cases, however, such a person would fall within the exception to the act relating to drug abusers whose current use of drugs prevents performance of employment duties or constitutes a direct threat to the safety or property of others.

Therefore, the Rehabilitation Act does not appear to pose a significant obstacle to drug testing in the workplace or to create any greater rights for workers who use drugs than would ordinarily exist under the U.S. Constitution and the other protections already discussed. Indeed, no court has found these "rights" to exist. The only clear protection offered by the Rehabilitation Act is for prior drug abusers who no longer use drugs. Under the act, they cannot be discriminated against as a class. However, because they have ended their drug abuse they would not suffer negative effects from testing; that is, they would not test positive.

Similar laws have been enacted in various states. New York and New Jersey expanded existing anti-discrimination laws to protect drug-dependent or alcohol-dependent employees who are in treatment.[87] California employers must provide "reasonable accommodation" to alcohol-dependent employees who participate voluntarily in a rehabilitation program. This includes allowing time off from work as long as no undue hardship results.[88]

New Jersey law further prohibits drug testing of job applicants until after an employment offer has been made.[89] Where such restrictions exist, application forms should include both a consent form authorizing a drug test and a statement expressly conditioning employment on successful completion of the test.[90]

Few if any state rehabilitation laws will protect current drug or alcohol abusers who refuse to seek treatment. Again, common sense dictates that employers consult with legal counsel on relevant state laws and their interpretation by the courts.

AVOIDING LEGAL PROBLEMS: A VIEW FROM THE COURTS

As noted above, the private employer is not bound by the federal constitutional restraints imposed upon the government employer. Nevertheless, private companies will be held accountable for failing to act reasonably in conducting employee drug testing or other drug-detection programs. This chapter began by pointing out the clash between evolving social attitudes and the laws as they affect drug testing. The private employer legally is entitled to do a great deal more than what may be accepted socially. However, because social attitudes can and do shape law and employer-employee relations, a wise employer will be sensitive to those attitudes in structuring a drug-testing program. If carried out with reasonableness and discretion, a testing program can satisfy both social and legal standards.

Threshold Decisions

There are two key threshold questions that businesses considering a drug-testing program should address. If a company can answer these questions persuasively, its workers in all probability will accept the company's testing program and policy and not file legal challenges.

The first question an employer must answer is: Why do I want to test? A company should be able to justify the decision to test by clearly showing employees *why* drug use cannot be tolerated. Would drug use cause an employee to be unfit for his or her job? Would drug use endanger either the safety of co-workers or the safety of the public? Does an employee hold a position of public trust? Few would question the right to test an airline pilot or railroad engineer, but keep in mind that some employees (the night janitor, the grocery store clerk) may be able to perform their jobs and perform them without endangering anyone's safety after smoking marijuana or using other illegal substances. Both the courts and arbitrators probably will be more supportive of testing if the employees affected are piloting an airplane or working around high-voltage wires than if they are bagging groceries. On the other hand, many companies take the position that illegal drug use by any of their employees affects health, safety, and productivity, and will not be tolerated. Reasoning in several court decisions supports this basis for action and these across-the-board policies may well be upheld.

An employer must also answer a second question: What do I do when I find that someone is using drugs? Before beginning testing, a company must develop clear procedures based upon a fully articulated, written policy for dealing with employees who test positive. These procedures must be *communicated clearly, enforced consistently, and applied fairly.* They should be based firmly on the principle that drug abuse affects the health and safety of all workers and that, where possible, drug abusers will be given assistance in overcoming their problem.

An employer must ensure that an employee substance-abuse program is reasonable. What follows are some features that might be included in such a program:

- Demonstrate the need for drug testing in the company; where possible, document a relationship between job performance and substance abuse.
- Develop a specific substance abuse policy and program in consultation with all parts of the company that may be affected. Union representatives, occupational health and safety personnel, security staff, personnel managers, legal advisers and, most important, top management all must be involved. Often companies have found it useful to bring in outside consultants to help identify problems and adopt a workable policy.
- Notify employees of the policy. Provide educational materials on the hazards of drug use. Tell employees in advance the penalties that will be imposed for specific violations. If necessary, modify private employment contracts and union contracts to reflect the company's substance abuse program.
- Train your supervisors to detect job-related problems and have them refer workers for evaluation by trained personnel. Do not have them diagnose aberrant behavior as substance abuse.

- Follow through. Do not let a substance abuse program become a "paper" policy.
- Test for substance abuse carefully. Hire a reputable laboratory. Confirm all positive test results with gas chromatography/mass spectrometry or equivalent methodologies and technologies. Make sure that those who administer the tests and perform laboratory analyses are qualified to do so.
- Notify employees and applicants of positive test results and provide them an opportunity to contest disciplinary actions taken on the basis of those results.
- Keep test results confidential. Do not release positive test results until their accuracy has been verified by a confirmatory test and, if possible, by corroborating evidence of substance abuse. Do not allow anyone who does not need to know have the results.
- Document improvements in the workplace that result from drug testing; for example, changes in absenteeism or work-related injuries.
- Consider setting up an employee assistance program or improving an existing one.

Elements of a Drug-Testing Program:
The Customs Service Example

The recent court case involving a union challenge to the Customs Service drug-testing program[91] provides a detailed analytical framework for evaluating other programs. While compliance with each of the factors set out in this particular case may not guarantee judicial support for an employer's drug abuse program, being aware of these principles may assure both employees and the courts that a fair and reasonable approach has been taken.

Highlights of the Program

The Customs Service program can be defined by its prominent characteristics:

- Limited to applicants for, and those seeking transfers to, jobs with direct involvement in the interdiction of illicit drugs, or responsibility for carrying firearms or access to classified information.
- Notification that the new position is contingent on successful completion of a drug test.
- Appointment scheduled for urinalysis *after* all other requirements for transfer have been met.
- No adverse consequences in current position for withdrawal from transfer application.
- Sealed listing of all current medications and exposure to illicit drugs in preceding thirty days. This list is not opened unless the urine test is positive.
- Specimen is produced in a restroom with an "observer" outside the

stall. The observer maintains the chain-of-custody procedures, including sealing, labeling, recording, coding and mailing the sample. The observer also is trained to be alert to signs of sample tampering.

- Laboratory maintains a tracking system and continues chain-of-custody procedures; uses appropriate screening tests and confirms all positive samples with GC/MS; reserves part of specimen for possible retesting.
- Employees may resubmit positive urine specimen to laboratory of their choice.

Scope and Manner

The Court of Appeals in the *von Raab* case upheld the Customs Service program of testing certain employees for drug use. In reviewing the Customs Service drug-testing program, the court considered the scope of the program and the manner in which it was administered. The Customs Service program was limited in scope to only certain employees (i.e., those seeking transfers to sensitive positions) and limited in terms of supervisory discretion in interpreting test results. The court approved of these limits because they left little room for the exercise of management discretion in areas where abuses of discretion are most likely to occur; namely, who takes the test and how the test results affect the employee. These limits are particularly important "when searches are permitted in the absence of individualized suspicion . . ." in order to protect reasonable expectations of privacy.[92]

Likewise, the manner in which the Customs Service program was administered limits intrusiveness. Tested employees are not observed, the test is scheduled in advance, and all other requirements for the transfer are approved prior to taking the drug test. The appeals court did not minimize the constitutional concerns involved, but rather weighed them in relation to other types of searches:

> The degree of privacy invasion, while serious enough to implicate the Fourth Amendment, is not as intrusive as an invasion of bodily integrity or of the home, nor do employees suffer the indignity of either strip or body cavity searches.[93]

The strict chain-of-custody procedures that were observed also weighed heavily in favor of the Customs Service program.[94]

Justification

Justification relates to the initial threshold question: Why do you want to test your employees? In the case of the Customs Service, the appeals court found the drug interdiction role of the Customs Service to be compelling justification for testing employees seeking to serve in sensitive jobs. The court noted that not only is job performance affected by drug use, but that it also "undermines public confidence in the integrity of the Service."[95]

In justifying a drug-testing program, employers should consider the purpose of their industry or type of business, the role of employees scheduled for testing, and the level of public trust in the industry or business. The Customs Service justified its program based on the need for public confidence, its role in intercepting illicit drug trade, the susceptibility of drug-using employees to blackmail, and the use of firearms by some of its agents.

Place

The court merely noted in one sentence that a private restroom is the most practicable location at which to obtain a specimen for testing.[96] Again, employers should be sensitive to the privacy expectations of employees and develop procedures that minimize any embarrassment or perceived indignity. Behavior indicating an attempt to subvert the testing process may justify greater intrusiveness in order to obtain accurate results.

Voluntariness

The Customs Service testing program was not required of all employees. Moreover, any employees who triggered the testing mechanism by seeking a "sensitive" job would not be penalized in their current position for refusal to take the test.[97] The court did not consider the inability to obtain the sought-after transfer to be a penalty.

Employment Relationship

This principle considers the Fourth Amendment protection afforded government employees and related limits on permissible searches by the government. The court noted that "the government cannot . . . undertake searches of its employees simply by making consent a condition of employment."[98] Specifically, the search must be a *reasonable* condition of employment; for example, "routine searches of paper bags as a condition of employment in a penitentiary."[99]

Furthermore, an employer need not wait for evidence of drug use to test for drugs. Where the nature of the job requires assurances that the responsible employee is drug free and where the drug test is reasonable and limited in scope, the court emphasized the rights of the government employer in what may well become the most quoted sentence of the Customs Service case:

> It is not unreasonable to set traps to keep foxes from entering hen houses even in the absence of evidence of prior vulpine intrusion or individualized suspicion that a particular fox has an appetite for chickens.[100]

Purpose of Search

As discussed earlier in another context, "the need for protection against governmental intrusion diminishes if the investigation is neither designed to enforce criminal laws nor likely to be used to bring criminal charges against the person investigated."[101] The Customs Service program served a purely administrative purpose. Additionally, the drug test results were not used or intended to be used to punish employees. Even so, the Customs Service had to demonstrate that the *need* for drug testing outweighed the intrusiveness of such a search.

Analogy to Regulated Industry

In certain highly regulated industries, legitimate expectations of privacy are diminished and employers may conduct certain reasonable searches in order to assure compliance with the regulations "without any degree of individualized suspicion."[102] The cases supporting these searches cover enforcement of housing and fire codes, liquor and gun sales, and nuclear power plant regulations.[103] More recently, a U.S. Appeals Court upheld drug testing of jockeys as valid since horse racing is a highly regulated industry with a strong interest in maintaining public confidence.[104]

The baseline question in this area is: What are the reasonable expectations of employees and applicants vis-à-vis the acceptability or tolerance of drug use? Again, compare the reasonable expectations of the grocery store clerk with those of the airline pilot.

Availability of Less Intrusive Measures

The question here is not limited simply to the availability of other means to obtain information about employee drug use, but includes rather the reasonableness and efficacy of these alternate sources. Do they provide a "basis on which to evaluate [the employees'] integrity and reliability should they be assigned to work in sensitive positions"?[105] Employers would do well to use less intrusive measures if they provide timely, accurate, and comparable information. Yet the Court of Appeals in the *McDonnell* vs. *Hunter* case held that random drug testing was the "least intrusive" means of accomplishing this goal.[106]

Effectiveness

The Customs Service case cautions that "no privacy invasions should be permitted unless some good end is served."[107] The union argued that the Customs Service program would allow drug users time to abstain from drugs to obtain a negative test result. The appeals court, however, noted that "[t]he risk of detection . . . may deter drug-using employees from seeking more sensitive positions."[108]

Employers should ask themselves if their existing or planned drug-testing program meets the needs for which it was designed. Unreasonable or over-reaching aspects of a program obviously are susceptible to legal challenge.

Recently, the Federal Aviation Administration's (FAA) drug testing of flight service specialists was upheld. The court, in citing its reasons for denying injunctive relief, outlined many of the same program elements as those in the Customs Service case:

• Appropriate advance notice of the testing program.

- Rehabilitative purpose of program (employees who test positive may enter a rehabilitation program and a reassignment to less critical work).
- Inclusion of drug test as part of existing periodic physical examination that includes urine specimen.
- Sensitive or critical nature of subject employees' responsibilities.
- Strict chain-of-custody.
- Use of pre-test questionnaire covering current drug use, which remains sealed unless confirmatory drug test is positive.
- Opportunity for retesting of specimen.
- Use of reliable test procedures including GC/MS confirmatory test.
- Use of least intrusive, most effective means.[109]

Noting these factors, the court agreed with the FAA that the legitimate privacy expectations of the flight service specialists were outweighed by "the national interests in air safety and the public's perception of safety."[110]

The drug-testing program that includes these elements will be most effective, not simply because it can withstand legal challenges but because the presence of these elements should increase the level of employee trust and cooperation. Likewise, public faith in and acceptance of drug-testing programs should be strengthened as more companies use these programs and document their effectiveness in terms of a safer and more productive workplace and improved public safety record.

UNRESOLVED QUESTIONS

Even the most carefully constructed drug-testing program can be the subject of legitimate debate in the areas of when the test is conducted (pre-employment, "for cause," random versus scheduled testing) and which categories of employees are tested ("sensitive" versus routine responsibilities). No one case provides across-the-board guidance in these areas. However, using the elements outlined thus far along with some caution and common sense, employers should be able to avoid pitfalls in these two areas.

Random Testing

The issue of random testing—that is, unannounced mandatory testing of all or a certain category of employees—has raised the largest concern in the entire drug-testing debate. This is entirely understandable. We are more concerned over someone losing his or her livelihood for illegal drug use than over rejection of a person who is applying for a position. We feel that people have a "right" to their jobs unless they commit some act that directly affects their work performance. Because of this notion, very few private or public employers randomly test workers for drug use. Those that do (airlines, bus companies, nuclear power plant operations) usually have a very clear reason for doing so.

The most important case in this area upheld random drug testing of correctional officers who had direct contact with inmates, even absent reasonable suspicion that illegal drugs had been used.[111] The court based its ruling on the types of duties performed by the employees and how the tests were conducted. In this case, guards who had regular contact with prisoners could be tested randomly for drugs as long as the tests were not performed in an "arbitrary or discriminatory" manner.[112] On the other hand, in the absence of regular contact with prisoners, safety and security concerns would not obviate the need for reasonable suspicion in order to perform drug tests. (A lower court specifically allowed pre-employment, periodic physical examinations and "for cause" testing.)[113]

An appeal of this case to the U.S. Supreme Court is expected. The progress of this case is worth noting, especially in terms of its impact on the Bush administration's proposal to drug-test government employees in "sensitive" positions.

The ruling here has limited application to industries outside of law enforcement and correctional institutions. This court, however, relied in part on the *Shoemaker* case upholding random urine testing of jockeys because of the "strong [state] interest in assuring the public of the integrity of the persons engaged in the horse racing industry."[114] The *McDonnell* court stated:

> We believe the state's interest in safeguarding the security of its correctional institutions is at least as strong as its interest in safeguarding the integrity of, and the public confidence in, the horse racing industry.[115]

This same analogy could be made to a variety of job categories in the transportation, nuclear power, and defense industries. First, however, the employer should return to the threshold question of "Why test?" and consider two additional questions here. Is *random* testing necessary to accomplish the purpose of a testing program? Is it the least intrusive, most effective method available?

Virginia's attorney general has offered an opinion that random drug testing of state employees, "including public safety personnel, would likely not be permissible."[116] Furthermore, "the legality of any [Virginia] drug testing program would depend on the particular circumstances of the *duties* of the employees and *how* the tests are conducted"[117] (emphasis added).

Private employers should be conservative in this area. Where random testing cannot be justified, employers should be prepared to document reasonable suspicion to conduct a drug test.

On the other hand, private (and government) employers seem to be on safe ground if their drug-testing programs include random testing of current employees who are in a rehabilitation program as a result of a positive drug test. The FAA program provided for observed random urine drug testing for one year following a positive finding. A second positive finding would result in reassignment and possible termination.

> This greater intrusion, however, is arguably justified since a positive urinalysis for prohibited substances may identify the employee as a substance abuser and establishes *reasonable suspicion* warranting more intrusive drug testing.[118] (Emphasis added.)

"Sensitive" versus Routine Jobs

Litigation regarding drug-testing programs has focused largely on government employees with job responsibilities affecting security or safety concerns. (A possible exception to this principle is the testing of jockeys and athletes, approved by the U.S. Third Circuit Court of Appeals.) Appropriately constructed testing of job applicants is generally accepted, as is testing of current employees where a reasonable suspicion for drug use exists. However, the validity of drug testing of current employees in the absence of reasonable suspicion seems to hinge on the kinds of responsibilities assigned to the employees subject to testing.

The FAA case provides some guidance here. Recall that the court upheld the FAA substance abuse control program that required employees in sensitive jobs to submit to urinalysis for drug testing as part of a periodic physical examination. One of the plaintiff's contentions was that flight service specialists do not perform sensitive or critical duties. The court disagreed and in so doing outlined general guidelines for evaluating sensitive jobs in the drug-testing context. These included:

- Degree of public trust in the industry.
- Importance of the job to the overall program.
- Level and degree of supervision.
- Risk factors involved.
- Reliance by other employees on information provided in making decisions affecting public safety.[119]

Obviously, the application of these criteria could result in a broad variety of results. Another word of caution: Avoid developing multiple sets of criteria for evaluating jobs. The court in the FAA case did not look favorably on the fact that the FAA classified flight service specialists as sensitive jobs for purposes of drug testing and as non-sensitive for purposes of personnel and retirement policies.[120]

STATE LEGISLATION

As more and more state legislatures respond to the problem of drugs in the workplace, new state laws will add to the issues and considerations discussed here. Some of these laws will serve to restrict or even prohibit an employer's ability to use drug testing as part of a substance-abuse prevention program. In fact, most state legislatures and courts that have considered drug testing "have set narrower testing guidelines than those sanctioned by federal courts or proposed by the Reagan administration for federal employees."[121] Parts of the above legal discussion may be rendered moot by such legislative proposals.

As of July 1987, more than thirty states were considering a variety of approaches to drug testing. Maine and Oregon are seeking to ban testing; Connecticut, Iowa, Montana, and Vermont have enacted laws that ban random testing and severely limit pre-employment testing; Massachusetts and New Jersey would allow "for cause" testing (*e.g.,* obvious impairment of job performance or existence of safety hazard). Utah has enacted a law that specifically permits employers to test current or prospective employees under certain conditions.

Additionally, employers must be aware of municipal and city ordinances related to drug testing. A San Francisco ordinance virtually prohibits random drug testing of any public or private employee.[122]

The American Civil Liberties Union has a strong interest in this area as well. An ACLU branch has drafted model legislation that would virtually ban the use of drug testing in the workplace. This proposed legislation, which has been introduced in Maryland, would also restrict testing of applicants for employment.[123]

CONCLUSION

Statistics abound on the costs of employee substance abuse in terms of decreased productivity, increased absenteeism, accidents at work, theft, higher health care premiums, and more union grievances. There are also costs that cannot be measured in dollars: the negative publicity suffered by affected companies; the damage to positions of public trust when a police officer or a corrections guard is using, or even rumored to be using, drugs; the lowered morale of nonabusers forced to work beside co-workers who are not pulling their own weight, but instead are endangering others' safety and committing crimes right in front of them. These realities make it relatively easy for most companies to answer the question: Why do I need to test for drugs? The more difficult the question is the second one: What do I do when I find out that someone is using drugs?

Assisting an employee to obtain treatment is almost always the better course of action than taking disciplinary action. Wise employers recognize the need to provide health assistance to impaired employees for purposes of sustaining employee morale and, as important, for economic reasons. While private employers have no legal obligations to rehabilitate their employees, it is almost always better, and less expensive, to keep an employee working than to find and train a replacement—who might also turn out to be a substance abuser.

Several services are available to industry today that can help companies handle drug and alcohol problems in a way that allows early intervention and effective treatment. This reduces absenteeism, prevents accidents, and makes for a healthier and safer workplace. Working through trained counselors, employers can improve the health of their employees and upgrade their job performance.

A carefully planned ..id implemented substance-abuse policy will help a company avoid both the problems of employee substance abuse and the employee dissatisfaction that results in legal action against the company. Judges and arbitrators increasingly are recognizing the costs of substance abuse in the workplace to employers, workers, and the economy. They will uphold measures designed to deal with the problem, including drug testing, when they are instituted in a reasonable manner. Barring restrictive legislation, employers who follow the above guidelines and have answered the questions "Why do I want to test?" and "What do I do when someone tests positive?" should be able to use drug testing effectively and legally.

NOTES

1. Executive Order 12564, Sept. 15, 1986.
2. *Id.*, Sections 1(c) and 3(a).
3. *American Medical News,* May 8, 1987, at 10.
4. *Time,* March 17, 1986, at 57.
5. The Presidential Commission on Organized Crime in its 1986 report has even suggested the usefulness of drug testing as a tool in reducing the demand for illegal drugs in this country. This chapter, however, will focus on the primary reasons for drug testing—protecting the health and safety of employees and improving the productivity of the work force.
6. *Time,* October 21, 1985, at 61.
7. *Washington Post,* May 5, 1986, at B8.
8. "Drug Use in Military Drops; Pervasive Testing Credited," *The New York Times,* April 23, 1987, at A17.
9. Some state constitutions, e.g., California, have a specific provision guaranteeing a "right to privacy." Private employers in these jurisdictions should determine whether the courts have applied this to drug-testing programs.
10. *Griswold* v. *Connecticut,* 381 U.S. 479, 483 (1965) ("the First Amendment has a penumbra where privacy is protected from governmental intrusion"); *Roe* v. *Wade,* 410 U.S. 113, 152 (1973) ("a right of personal privacy, or a guarantee of certain areas or zones of privacy, does exist under the Constitution. In varying contexts, the Court or individual Justices have, indeed, found at least the roots of that right in the First Amendment, . . . in the Fourth and Fifth Amendments, . . . in the penumbras of the Bill of Rights, . . . guaranteed by the first section of the Fourteenth Amendment." (Citations omitted.) [Note Supreme Court case (Ga. 1986) relating to homosexual acts not being protected.]
11. "The right to possess and use marijuana in one's own home is not and

cannot be classified as a fundamental right protected by a constitutional zone of privacy." *Louisiana Affiliate of the Nat'l Org. for the Reform of Marijuana Laws v. Guste,* 380 F. Supp. 404, 409 (E.D. La. 1974), *aff'd.* 511 F.2d 1400 (5th Cir. 1975), *cert. denied,* 423 U.S. 867 (1975).

12. Officials of the American Civil Liberties Union and the Legal Action Center, both proponents of severe restrictions on drug testing, acknowledge that such constitutional protections do not apply to private employers. *Washington Post,* May 9, 1985, at D1. Testimony of Paul N. Samuels, Executive Vice President, the Legal Action Center, before the House Select Committee on Narcotics Abuse and Control, May 7, 1984.

13. "The right of the people to be secure in their persons, houses, papers, and effects, against unreasonable searches and seizures, shall not be violated, and no Warrants shall issue, but upon probable cause, supported by Oath or affirmation, and particularly describing the place to be searched, and the persons or things to be seized." U.S. CONST. amend. IV.

14. *Turner v. Fraternal Order of Police,* 500 A.2d 1005 (App. D.C. 1985).

15. *Id.* at 1008.

16. *Allen v. City of Marietta,* 601 F. Supp. 482 (N.D. Ga. 1985).

17. *Id.* at 491.

18. *Nat'l Assn. of Air Traffic Specialists (NAATS) v. Dole,* No. A87-073 (D. Alaska March 27, 1987), at 3.

19. *Division 241 Amalgamated Transit Union (AFL-CIO) v. Suscy,* 538 F.2d 1264 (7th Cir. 1976), *cert. denied,* 429, U.S. 1029 (1976).

20. *Division 241, Amalgamated Transit Union (AFL-CIO) v. Suscy,* 405 F. Supp. 750, 751-752 (N.D. Ill. 1975).

21. *Division 241 Amalgamated Transit Union (AFL-CIO) v. Suscy,* 538 F.2d 1264, 1267 (7th Cir. 1976), *cert. denied,* 429 U.S. 1029 (1976).

22. *Shoemaker v. Handel,* 795 F.2d 1136 (3rd Cir. 1986).

23. *McDonell v. Hunter,* 809 F.2d 1302 (8th Cir. 1987).

24. *Id.* at 1308.

25. *National Treasury Employees Union (NTEU) v. von Raab,* 816 F.2d 170 (5th Cir. 1987), *stay denied,* ___U.S.___, 107 S.Ct. 2479 (1987). Decision upheld 109 S.Ct. 1384 (1989).

26. *Id.* at 173, 179.

27. *Lovvorn v. City of Chattanooga, Tenn.,* 647 F. Supp. 875, 879 (E.D. Tenn. 1986).

28. *Id.* at 882.

29. *Id.* at 882–883.

30. *Fraternal Order of Police v. City of Newark,* 524 A.2d 430 (N.J. Super. Ct. App. Div. 1987).

31. *Id.* at 437.

32. Even with its limited authority to confirm drug and alcohol use, the Federal Railroad Administration has stated that between 1975 and 1984 alcohol or drug use played a causal role in, or materially affected the severity of, at least 48 injuries and $34.4 million in damages. Testimony of John H. Riley, Administrator, Federal Railroad Administration, before the House Select Committee on Narcotics Abuse and Control, May 7, 1986.

33. *Brotherhood of Locomotive Engineers v. Burlington Northern Railroad Co.,* No. CV-84-213-GF (D. Mont. 1984).

34. *Id.* at 4.

35. *Shell Oil Co.* v. *Oil, Chemical and Atomic Workers,* 84-1 Lab. Arb. Awards (CCH) ¶3101 (1983) (Brisco, Arb.).

36. *Id.* at 3104.

37. *NAATS* v. *Dole,* No. A87-073 (D. Alaska March 27, 1987); *NTEU* v. *von Raab,* 816 F.2d 170 (5th Cir. 1987) *stay denied,* ____U.S.____, 107 S.Ct. 2479 (1987).

38. Banzhaf, "How to Make Drug Tests Pass Constitutional Muster," 2 EMPLOYEE TESTING AND THE LAW, Feb. 1987, at 1.

39. *Id.* at 3.

40. *NTEU* v. *von Raab,* 816 F.2d 170, 179.

41. *Id.*

42. The federal government is bound by the Fifth Amendment, which provides: "No person shall . . . be deprived of life, liberty, or property, without due process of law." U.S. CONST. amend V. "[N]or shall any State deprive any person of life, liberty, or property, without due process of law." U.S. CONST. amend. XIV. §1.

43. *Hester* v. *City of Milledgeville,* 598 F. Supp. 1456 (M.D. Ga. 1984), *aff'd & rev'd in part* 777 F.2d 1492 (11th Cir. 1986). The appellate court held that the city could order employees to take a polygraph if, among other conditions, the results of the test would not be used as the sole ground for disciplinary action. The court left open the possibility that, under certain circumstances, disciplinary action based on a polygraph examination would not violate due process requirements.

44. *Smith* v. *State,* 250 Ga. 438, 298 S.E.2d 482 (1983).

45. *NTEU* v. *von Raab,* 816 F.2d 170 (5th Cir. 1987), *stay denied,* ____ U.S.____,107 S.Ct. 2479 (1987).

46. *Id.* at 174.

47. *Id.* at 173.

48. *Id.* at 181.

49. *Id.* at 181–182.

50. *Spence* v. *Farrier,* 807 F.2d 753, 756 (8th Cir. 1986).

51. *California* v. *Trombetta,* 467 U.S. 479 (1984).

52. *Id.* at 490 n.10.

53. *NAATs* v. *Dole,* No. A87-073 (D. Alaska March 27, 1987) at 68. Additionally, in January, 1987, the FDA issued more stringent labeling requirements for manufacturers of urine tests. The required labeling states in part: "All positive test results should be confirmed by an independent and more specific method . . . [GC/MS] is the confirmatory method of choice."

54. *See* Carr, *Employer Use of the "Lie Detector": The Arbitration Experience,* 1984 LAB. L.J. 701, 702-3.

55. *Id.; see also* 3 J. WEINSTEIN, EVIDENCE ¶607[04] for case survey.

56. *See e.g., Glen Manor Home for the Jewish Aged* v. *Union of Hosp. and Health Care Employees,* 85-1 LAB. ARB. AWARDS (CCH) ¶3139, 3141-2 (1984).

57. *Time,* March 17, 1986, at 61.

58. *New Orleans Public Service* v. *Masaracchia,* 464 So.2d 866 (La. Ct. App. 1985).

59. *Id.* at 868.

60. Crown Zellerbach and United Paperworkers, Local 752, FMCX Case 86K/09162, as noted in *Employee Testing and the Law,* April, 1987 at 7.

61. *Banks* v. *Federal Aviation Admin.*, 687 F.2d 92 (5th Cir. 1982) (the FAA allowed a laboratory to throw away samples before employee could independently inspect and test them).

62. *Harvey* v. *Chicago Transit Auth.*, No. 83-C-9074, slip op. (N.D. Ill. 1984) (involving disciplinary action against a Chicago bus driver).

63. *Pittard* v. *Four Seasons Motor Inn*, 688 P.2d 333 (N.M. Ct. App. 1984).

64. Breach of this duty not only may constitute negligence, but may be a violation of certain laws. For example, the Occupational Safety and Health Act requires that an employer "shall furnish to each of his employees employment and a place of employment which are free from recognized hazards that are causing or are likely to cause death or serious physical harm to his employees." 29 U.S.C. §654(a)(2). A substance-impaired co-worker operating heavy and/or dangerous machinery could present such a hazard.

65. *Id.*

66. *Time,* March 17, 1986, at 53.

67. *UAW* v. *General Dynamics*, ____F.2d____ (D.C. Cir. April 14, 1987).

68. "Negligent Hiring Claims Take Off," A.B.A.J., May 1, 1987, at 72-73.

69. *Triblo* v. *Quality Clinical Laboratories*, No. 82-226166-CZ (Mich. Ct. App. filed July 15, 1982; plaintiffs Chase and Medina withdrew after settlement reached). See, also footnote 53 re new FDA labeling requirements.

70. *Jones* v. *McKenzie*, 628 F. Supp. 1500, 1505-1506 (D.D.C. 1986).

71. *McCleod* v. *City of Detroit*, No. 83-CV-2163-DT (E.D. Mich. 1985).

72. *Ivy* v. *Damon Clinical Laboratory*, slip op. (Tenn. Ct. App. 1984).

73. *Houston Belt & Terminal Ry. Co.* v. *Wherry*, 548 S.W.2d 743 (Tex. Civ. App. 1976).

74. *Brotherhood of Locomotive Engineers* v. *Burlington Northern Railroad Co.*, 620 F. Supp. 173 (D. Mont. 1985).

75. *B. Green & Co.* v. *Warehouse Employers Union*, 71 Lab. Arb. (BNA) 685 (1978) (Cushman, Arb.).

76. *See, e.g.,* Dufek, Underhill, "Arbitration Can Thwart Employer No-Drug Policy," *Legal Times,* March 18, 1985, at 21.

77. 42 U.S.C. §290ee-1.

78. 29 U.S.C. §701 *et seg.* This statute has a potentially broad impact on private employers because of the large number of companies who do work under government contracts.

79. *See* 29 C.F.R. §32.3, 43 Op. Att'y. Gen. 12 (1977).

80. *Davis* v. *Bucher*, 451 F. Supp. 791, 795-96 (E.D. Pa. 1978).

81. 29 U.S.C. §706(7)(B).

82. *See McCleod* v. *City of Detroit*, No. 83-CV-2163-DT (E.D. Mich. 1985) (holding that persons removed from employment as city fire fighters after testing positive for marijuana use were not "handicapped individuals" protected by the Rehabilitation Act).

83. 29 U.S.C. §706(7)(B).

84. 29 C.F.R. §32.3.

85. *See Jasany* v. *United States Postal Service*, 755 F.2d 1244 (6th Cir. 1985); *E.E. Black, Ltd.* v. *Marshall*, 497 F. Supp. 1088 (D. Hawaii 1980).

86. *McCleod* v. *City of Detroit*, No. 83-CV-2163-DT (E.D. Mich. 1985).

87. Aron, *Drug Testing: The Employer's Dilemma*, 1987 LAB. L.J. 157, 164.

88. *Id.*

89. N.J. Admin. Code tit. 13:13-2.4(e).

90. Aron, *Drug Testing: The Employer's Dilemma*, 1987 LAB. L.J. 157, 164.

91. *NTEU* v. *von Raab*, 816 F.2d 170 (5th Cir. 1987), *stay denied*, _____ U.S._____, 107 S.Ct. 2479 (1987). U.S. Supreme Court has since affirmed the Customs Service program. 109 S.Ct. 1384 (1989).

92. *Id.* at 177.

93. *Id.*

94. *Id.* at 181.

95. *Id.* at 178.

96. *Id.*

97. *Id.*

98. *Id.* at 179.

99. *Id.*

100. *Id.*

101. *Id.*

102. *Id.*

103. *Camera* v. *Municipal Court*, 387 U.S. 523 (1967) (upholding warrantless searches of residences without probable cause to believe that housing code violations existed); *See* v. *City of Seattle*, 387 U.S. 541 (1967) (warrant required to conduct administrative inspections of private commercial premises to ensure compliance with municipal fire code, but no requirement for probable cause); *Colonnade Catering Corp.* v. *U.S.*, 397 U.S. 72 (1970) (upholding warrantless inspections of liquor dealers' premises for purpose of ensuring compliance with federal law regulating liquor industry); *United States* v. *Biswell*, 406 U.S. 311 (1972) (upholding warrantless inspections of gun dealers' storerooms for purpose of ensuring compliance with federal Gun Control Act); and *Rushton* v. *Nebraska Public Power District*, 653 F. Supp. 1510 (D. Neb. 1987) (upholding mandatory drug testing without individualized suspicion of nuclear power plant employees with unescorted access to secure facilities).

104. *Shoemaker* v. *Handel*, 795 F.2d 1136 (3d Cir. 1986), *cert. denied*, _____U.S. 107 S.Ct. 577 (1986).

105. *NTEU* v. *von Raab*, 816 F.2d 170, 180 (5th Cir. 1987), *stay denied*, _____ U.S. _____, 107 S.Ct. 2479 (1987).

106. *McDonell* v. *Hunter*, 809 F.2d 1302 (8th Cir. 1987).

107. *NTEU* v. *von Raab*, 816 F.2d 170, 180 (5th Cuirc. 1987), *stay denied*, _____ U.S. _____, 107 S.Ct. 2479 (1987).

108. *Id.*

109. *NAATS* v. *Dole*, No. A87-073 (D. Alaska March 27, 1987).

110. *Id.* at 63.

111. *McDonell* v. *Hunter*, 809 F.2d 1302 (8th Cir. 1987).

112. *Id.* at 1303.

113. *Id.* at 1302.

114. *Shoemaker* v. *Handel*, 795 F.2d 1136, 1142 (3d Cir. 1986), *cert. denied*, _ U.S._____, 107 S.Ct. 577 (1986).

115. *McDonell* v. *Hunter*, 809 F.2d 1302, 1308 (8th Cir. 1987).

116. "Random drug tests unlikely by State of Virginia," 2 EMPLOYEE TESTING AND THE LAW, April 1987, at 4.

117. *Id.*

118. *NAATS* v. *Dole*, No. A87-073 (D. Alaska March 27, 1987), at 11.

119. *Id.* at 48.

120. *Id.* at 45-46.
121. *Washington Post,* June 19, 1987, at A4.
122. San Francisco Ordinance No. 527-85 (1985). Testing of other employees is limited to situations where the employer has reasonable grounds to believe the employee's faculties are impaired on the job, the impairment presents a "clear and present danger" to the employee or others, and the employer provides an opportunity, at employer expense, to have any blood or urine samples tested by an independent laboratory and to rebut or explain the results of any test.
123. Maryland House of Delegates Bill No. 1672 (February 7, 1987).

9

Ethical Issues in Drug Testing

BERNARD LO

College athletes, air traffic controllers, and railway workers have been asked to take drug tests. Concern about drug abuse in America and economic losses attributable to drug use by workers have spurred the growth of drug-testing programs. According to the White House, one in six federal workers uses illicit drugs regularly and 44 percent of new employees have used drugs in the previous year (Holden, 1987). Employers lose an estimated $60 million to $100 million annually because of absenteeism, lower productivity, turnover, and medical costs related to drug use by employees (Polankoff, 1987). Among Fortune 500 companies, an estimated 40 percent had urine drug-screening programs in 1986, compared to 18 percent the previous year (Hoyt et al., 1987). Despite such increases in drug testing, difficult questions remain concerning when it is appropriate. The ethical principles that guide medical practice (Lo, 1988; Beauchamp & Childress, 1983; Englehardt, 1986)—autonomy, nonmalefi cence, beneficence, and justice—should also direct decisions about drug testing.

ETHICAL PRINCIPLES

Autonomy

According to the principle of autonomy, or respect for persons, individuals should be allowed to determine their own course of action in accordance with their values and plans. For example, competent, informed people have the right to make decisions about their bodies and health care and to refuse tests and treatments recommended by their physicians (President's Commission for the Study of Ethical Problems, 1982). Respecting autonomy is a strong ethical duty. Philosophers have also argued that it is the very basis of a secular moral community (Englehardt, 1986, pp. 39–49). In addition, values such as privacy, liberty, individuality, and independence are deeply rooted in American society.

190

Respect for autonomy is closely linked to the right of privacy, the right to be left alone and to be free of government interference or bodily intrusion. Privacy has also been characterized as being protected from unwanted access by others, including physical access, personal information, or attention (Bok, 1982). People naturally want to guard against others touching their bodies, learning too much about them, or simply paying too much attention to them. Privacy and liberty are so highly prized that the U.S. Constitution and the courts have restricted searches, seizures, and detentions in criminal investigations. The implicit value judgment is that it is preferable to let some criminals go free rather than to infringe on the autonomy of innocent citizens (Kamisar, 1987). Courts have ruled that testing of urine for drugs constitutes a search under the Fourth Amendment (Glantz, 1989).

Drug testing may be regarded as an infringement of autonomy because it violates privacy. Privacy needs to be judged from the point of view of the person being tested, not from the point of view of those doing the testing. Drug tests are run on specimens of blood or urine. Most individuals being tested regard venipuncture as a bodily invasion. Patients accept it when a medical test is being conducted for their own benefit, but the same level of invasion may not be acceptable for other purposes. Providing a urine sample is less invasive than having blood drawn—there is no bodily touching or needlestick. But urinating into a container on demand may be considered embarrassing and demeaning, particularly when the purpose is questionable. Furthermore, to prevent cheating, the subject tested may be observed and listened to while urinating. Historians have pointed out that for centuries people have expected that intimate bodily functions will not be observed by others (Thomas, 1989).

Drug testing in the workplace can also be considered to violate privacy because workers may feel that their lives outside the workplace are no business of the employer, as long as they perform their jobs satisfactorily. In this regard, urine tests for drugs may actually be *more* invasive than blood tests because they provide information about drug use days to weeks before the test. Workers may object because such information will still be obtained even though the drug could no longer affect job performance. They may wish to have control over personal information about themselves and to determine to whom such information is revealed. Such control is essential to the concept of privacy.

Drug testing and infringements on privacy are justified, of course, if people consent to testing. But consent is valid only when targeted individuals have a real choice to decline testing. For example, advocates of drug testing in sports may argue that athletes who do not want to be tested can choose not to participate on the team or in the competition. But athletes committed to excelling in their sport may have little choice but to compete on the terms dictated. Athletes may have no alternatives to joining a team or entering a tournament if they want top-level competition. Furthermore, for some athletes, sport may be a livelihood or a potential career rather than merely a recreation, so that the issue is one of workplace drug testing.

An employer may defend a policy of testing all job applicants or workers by arguing that those who do not wish to be tested can seek employment elsewhere. But applicants or workers may not really have alternatives, unless they are willing to accept reduced wages, geographical dislocation, or a lower-level position not commensurate with their experience or training. While the worker or applicant may assent to testing, the choice may not be a truly autonomous decision.

Consent to drug testing may also be constrained by suspicions about those who do not agree to testing. "Voluntary" testing in which it is implied that those who are not tested have something to hide is not truly voluntary. If people believe that they must prove they are innocent by taking a drug test, they are not free to refuse testing. For example, when the San Francisco 49ers football team instituted voluntary drug testing, one player said that he was afraid to object to the test because resistance might seem like an admission of guilt (Cohn, 1987). Suggestions that if people have nothing to hide, they would agree to testing contradict the usual American presumption that people are innocent until proven guilty.

On the other hand, arguments based on autonomy have also been used to justify drug testing. First, it makes little sense to speak of the autonomy of people who are incapable of informed, free choices (President's Commission, 1982, pp. 55–68). Those with severe dementia or psychosis are considered incompetent to make decisions about their medical care. Similarly, it could be argued that chronic drug users are incapable of making informed choices about drug testing because their judgment is impaired. Indeed, their actions may be driven by physical or psychological addiction rather than determined by their true character or values. Drug testing might even enhance autonomy in the long run by motivating individuals to seek treatment to free them from dependency on drugs. This line of reasoning, however, would support only selective testing of individuals whose job performance is impaired, not universal testing. It cannot be assumed that *all* workers lack the capacity to make decisions about drug testing and treatment. Furthermore, it may not be acceptable to curtail the autonomy of those who are competent in order to detect those whose competence may be impaired.

A second argument in support of drug testing appeals to the autonomy of employers. (Note, however, that it does not make sense to talk about autonomy of large corporations in the same way that we talk about the autonomy of individuals.) Employers have an interest in reducing worker absenteeism and health care costs and increasing productivity. It can be argued that they should be allowed to run their business according to their own values and preferences. However, one person's autonomy is always limited by the need to respect the autonomy of others. People are not permitted to exercise their own autonomy in ways that infringe on the autonomy of others or that violate other moral duties. In general, economic interests do not justify overriding the autonomy of other people.

Nonmaleficence

The principle of nonmaleficence requires people to refrain from injuring others or to prevent harm to others (Beauchamp & Childress, 1983, pp. 106–147). In some situations, society has determined that the duty to prevent harm to third parties overrides the duty to respect autonomy and privacy. For example, cases of infectious diseases such as tuberculosis must be reported to public health officials. The justification is that contacts of infected individuals may not realize they are at risk for infection. Unless such contacts are notified of their risk and advised to seek treatment, they may be seriously harmed (Lo, 1988). For similar reasons, society restricts automobile driving of those who have conditions causing marked confusion or blackout spells because they may harm others. Testing for alcohol intoxication is required by law by when actions of the driver suggest that he or she is enebriated.

In drug testing, the dilemma is what risk to others justifies overriding the privacy of a worker? Several levels of risk need to be distinguished, which have decreasing strength as justifications for drug testing in the workplace. First, if harm to others has already occurred, as through an accident, drug testing of the responsible worker is clearly appropriate as part of a comprehensive investigation. Such testing, however, may seem too late in that innocent people have already been harmed.

Second, there may be reasonable evidence that a worker's job performance is impaired by drug abuse and that the safety of third parties may be compromised. Again, drug testing would seem justified. While individuals have a right to jeopardize their own health or safety, they do not have the right to place others at risk (Gaylin, 1987). For example, drug testing would be justified if a police officer, airplane pilot, or physician, who has responsibility for the safety or health of others, showed evidence of impaired performance or judgment. Other workers might imperil their colleagues if their performance were impaired.

However, in many jobs, there are no evaluations of a worker's performance that might legitimately trigger drug testing. Indeed, some drug-testing programs may be envisioned as substitutes for more direct evaluations of job performance.

Third, there may be evidence that within an occupation responsible for the safety of others, there is widespread drug abuse. For example, drug testing of railroad workers was imposed by the federal government because many railway workers got drugs on the job and 23 percent were problem drinkers (Kamisar, 1987). This rationale for testing is less persuasive than evidence of impaired performance by an individual worker.

Finally, the very nature of the work may be claimed as a reason for drug testing, even if there is no evidence of impaired individual performance or drugs problems in the occupation. Thus, some might argue that any workers who might jeopardize the safety or well-being of others should undergo drug testing. Such occupations might include government officials, airplane pilots, and nurses. The potential list of occupations to be tested might be very long indeed, and it would be difficult to justify testing some groups but not others. Obviously the latter justifications are weaker than the former. The need to prevent harm to third parties more clearly outweighs the need to respect the privacy of workers in the first two situations.

The duty of nonmaleficence is owed those who are tested as well as to third parties who may be harmed. The person tested may be inappropriately harmed in several ways. False-positive tests may occur, because of laboratory error, specimen labeling, or random variation. The predictive value of drug testing should be acceptable. (The positive predictive value is the probability that a person who tests positive actually has used drugs.) Critics have pointed out that a positive urine screening test is more likely to be falsely positive when the prior probability (the likelihood that the individual had used drugs before the test results were available) is low (Polankoff, 1987). Indeed, in some populations, the accuracy of the tests may be so low that they provide no useful information. The Office of Technology Assessment projects that if the prevalence of drug use is 2 percent, the predictive value of a positive urine screening test is only 16 percent (Miike, 1987). In other words, five out of every six positive tests are false positives. Using the same assumptions about the accuracy of testing, we can calculate that if the prevalence of drugs use is 16 percent (as estimated by the White House), the positive predictive value would still be only 64 percent. Those labeled as drug users would suffer tremendous harm if positive urine assays were not confirmed by more specific confirmatory tests.

The proficiency of the laboratory doing the testing must also be checked. Deficiencies in quality control may lead to inaccurate test results. On blinded proficiency testing of fifty laboratories, the false-positive rate was 1.3 percent (Davis, Hawks, & Blanke, 1988). Most laboratories do not undergo blinded proficiency testing. While their accuracy is unknown, it is probably lower than values reported for laboratories willing to participate in blinded proficiency testing.

Harm to those tested can also be minimized by careful attention to testing procedures. Intrusions on privacy should be minimized when urine samples are obtained. The confidentiality of test results must be maintained. Only those who have a legitimate need to know should be told of an employee's test results, and safeguards should be established to prevent further dissemination of results without sound reason. Test results must be interpreted properly. A confirmed positive test means only that the worker had used drugs; it is not necessarily evidence of drug abuse or impaired work performance. Furthermore, assays may detect drugs legitimately prescribed by physicians or medications available over the counter without prescription, as well as illicit drugs.

Beneficence

The principle of beneficence enjoins us to act to benefit others. It is, however, a weaker moral obligation than the principle of nonmaleficence. There is no common agreement on what is good, how much good ought to be done, or to whom such good is owed (Englehardt, 1986, pp. 66–79). Moreover, a duty to take steps to benefit others would lead to open-ended and impractical responsibilities (Beauchamp & Childress, 1983, pp. 148–158). Thus while benefiting others may be praiseworthy and virtuous, it is not obligatory.

Because beneficence is a relatively weak moral duty, it does not justify drug-testing programs. It is sometimes argued that drug testing is legitimate because it identifies workers who need help or who might harm themselves. Philosophers use the term *paternalism* for overruling an individual's actions or wishes in order to benefit that person (Childress, 1982; Englehardt, 1986, pp. 279–284). Paternalistic actions generally limit the person's liberty or autonomy. Most commentators reject paternalism if the person is competent, informed, and not coerced. Thus, although improving the health and lifestyle of workers is a worthwhile goal, it does not justify limiting their autonomy and privacy.

Paternalism can be justified, however, when the subject is incompetent, uninformed, or coerced (technically called *weak paternalism*). In these situations, there is no conflict between beneficence and autonomy because the person is not capable of autonomous action. Hence, justifications of weak paternalism would support testing workers who have shown impaired job performance that could endanger themselves. These arguments, however, would not justify universal drug testing of all workers in risky jobs.

The principle of beneficence also requires that the benefits of testing be proportionate to the harm it might cause. For there to be *any* benefit from drug testing, test results must be accurate and reliable. For the benefits to be proportionate to the harm caused by intrusions on privacy, there must be important social benefits that cannot be attained without testing. Furthermore, drug-testing programs might benefit those tested by attempting to counsel and rehabilitate individuals who test positive, particularly before terminating employment.

Justice

The principle of justice or fairness obliges us to give all people what they are due. To be fair, drug testing should observe procedural safeguards. The protocol for testing should be explicit and publicized before testing is initiated. Workers should know under what circumstances testing will be triggered. Precautions must be taken to avoid incorrect identification of specimens, and an appeals process should be established and publicized.

Justice also requires that the benefits, burdens, and costs of testing be distributed equitably. Those who benefit from testing are generally not the same individuals who bear the burdens of testing. Employers and third parties may benefit from testing, whereas employees who are tested suffer invasion of privacy and bear the risks of false-positive tests, termination of employment, and social stigma. Justice also requires that drug-testing programs reduce to acceptable levels the possible harm to those who undergo screening for the benefit of others.

Furthermore, justice requires that similar classes of persons be treated similarly. We should not discriminate inappropriately with regard to who is tested and what substances are tested. For instance, if drug testing were deemed appropriate for nurses whose impaired performance could put patients at risk, then fairness would dictate that physicians also be tested. The principle of justice also highlights the inconsistency of drug programs that do not test for alcohol, even though alcoholism is a major cause of work-related accidents. It is difficult to test for alcohol because it and its metabolites are rapidly cleared from the body. Furthermore, alcohol is a legal drug that is widely used without endangering others. The director of the Alcohol, Drug Abuse and Mental Health Administration called alcohol a "red herring," saying that the government could not very well take sanctions against every sailor coming back tipsy from shore leave (Polankoff, 1987). The implication is that a drug program should not concern itself with alcohol use that does not impair work performance. But then fairness requires that testing for other drugs should also be linked to impaired job performance.

In addition, justice mandates that the resources allocated to drug-screening programs be proportionate to benefits attained and to the resources available for other meritorious programs. For instance, drug-testing programs should be compared to alternative measures to achieve the goals of preventing harm to third parties or reducing illicit drug use. Such alternatives would include education, counseling, voluntary drug-treatment programs, and direct testing of job performance in workers who might endanger others.

RESOLVING CONFLICTS

Ethical principles and duties may conflict with each other. For example, the duty to protect the autonomy of individuals undergoing testing clashes with the duty to prevent harm to third parties. Such conflicts raise dilemmas because there are cogent reasons to support each obligation. While

controversy is unavoidable, some general comments for resolving conflicting duties and interests can be offered.

Litigation

While litigation offers an approach to resolving such conflicts, it may not
always be the best approach. In American society the courts are the final
arbiters; lawsuits can always yield a decision about whether drug testing
is appropriate in a given situation. But using the courts to resolve disputes
may be time-consuming, particularly if the appeals process is prolonged.
Because a court decision addresses only a particular set of circumstances,
the common law may be slow to fashion guidelines on drug testing. In
addition, regulations, requirements, or court decisions may apply only in
certain circumstances. Regulations and decisions regarding federal employees may not apply to private businesses that do not have government
contracts (Council on Scientific Affairs, 1987). Furthermore, litigation
may polarize the parties in the suit. Employers and employees who are
involved in adversarial court proceedings may find it difficult later to cooperate in the workplace. Finally, the question of whether it is legal to
test employees for drugs is not the only question that needs to be addressed. The law sets minimum standards and allows much room for discretion. Even if drug testing is legally permissible, it may not be morally
obligatory or commendable. The law also does not address the question
of whether a particular drug-testing program is a good one, rather than a
minimally acceptable one.

Ranking Ethical Principles

Another approach to resolving disputes about drug testing is to determine
which ethical principles or duties take priority over others. However,
there is no complete ranking or ordering of ethical duties or principles
that is universally accepted or that applies to all circumstances. Nevertheless, three priorities among ethical principles are generally accepted in
American society, as we have already suggested.

First, autonomy is granted great respect in American culture because
values like independence, liberty, individuality, and privacy are highly
prized. The general presumption, the starting point for debate, is that
violations of privacy are *prima facie* inappropriate and require justification. Although there might be situations in which autonomy may be
overridden, the burden of proof is generally on those who would violate
autonomy.

Second, nonmaleficence may take priority over autonomy. Maintaining
privacy and individual liberty do not justify endangering the safety of unknowing third parties. Thus, not only is drug testing permissible when
workers endanger others, but employers have a positive obligation to

identify such impaired workers and prevent them from harming others. Drug testing may be an important aspect of such a program.

Third, beneficence is usually subordinate to autonomy. Paternalistic actions can be justified only in certain limited circumstances. The prospect of benefit to the worker who receives treatment for drug abuse is not an acceptable reason for involuntary drug testing.

Although people may agree on these priorities among conflicting ethical principles, they may disagree over how to interpret those priorities or principles in a particular case. For example, most people would agree that overriding worker autonomy is acceptable when there is a reasonable suspicion of drug use and the worker presents a serious danger to third parties. But terms such as "reasonable" and "serious" are ambiguous and subject to different interpretations. People who agree on the general rule may disagree over what constitutes reasonable suspicion or serious danger. For example, chronic lateness, absenteeism, and repeated episodes of using excessive physical force would generally be considered reasonable grounds for suspecting that a police officer was impaired, possibly because of drug use. Similarly, an airplane pilot or neurosurgeon with poor coordination threatens the lives of passengers or patients. Less clear-cut cases, however, may be controversial.

Discussions about drug testing may overlook the problems in defining standards for work performance. Suppose a telephone operator at a police station or medical clinic does not recognize that a call involves an emergency case and treats it as a routine one. Suppose further that that particular day was unusually busy and that the situation was unusual. Does such an episode warrant drug testing? Do several such incidents? If so, how many? Furthermore, people in different roles might interpret such an incident differently. A citizen, politician, or patient advocate might be concerned that future similar episodes of poor judgment or delay might jeopardize public safety. On the other hand, the police chief or clinic director, concerned about adverse publicity, might minimize the gravity of the incident. A union leader might be more interested in additional staffing or better training than in investigating an individual worker. Thus, even after we agree on general rules about drug testing, controversy may continue over how to interpret and implement them.

Utilitarianism

One philosophical approach looks not at the priorities among conflicting ethical principles but to the consequences of actions. Utilitarian ethical systems determine whether actions are right or wrong by examining their consequences. They would have us act in ways that maximize the total social benefit relative to the total costs incurred and harm done. Utilitarianism, however, can be subjected to several serious criticisms. First, it may be difficult to compare both the benefit and the harm of different drug-testing policies. One drug program may offer both more benefit and more harm than another program or no program at all. Second, looking at total benefit and harm overlooks how these are distributed among different individuals. As we have indicated, the people who benefit from testing are not the same ones who bear the risks. It is difficult to agree on how to balance the benefit to one group against the harm to another. Third, utilitarian calculations of harm and benefit may overlook long-term and indirect consequences of actions. For instance, mandatory drug programs may give workers the message that they are under suspicion, not to be trusted, and in an adversarial position with management. Not respecting workers as people may decrease profits for the employer in the long run because workers who feel respected may be more satisifed and productive.

Finally, respect for liberty and privacy of all people may be eroded by acceptance of drug testing that violates the privacy and liberty of selected individuals in certain situations. The danger is that if we accept minor violations of privacy and liberty in one instance, we may be more willing to accept greater violations in subsequent situations. Thus, utilitarian calculations may not be appropriate when dealing with rights, such as the right to be free of unreasonable searches and seizures. Implicit in the concept of rights is that they should be overridden only for very weighty reasons. Rights should not be violated for benefits that are uncertain, controversial, or minor or which can be achieved by alternative means.

GUIDELINES FOR DRUG-TESTING PROGRAMS

The controversy over drug testing is likely to continue, stimulated by growing concern over drug abuse in the United States as well as concern for the competitiveness of American products in world markets. We suggest several ethical guidelines for deciding whether a drug-testing program is appropriate.

First, the goal of testing must be acceptable. Preventing serious physical harm to unsuspecting third parties justifies drug testing of individuals whose job performance is impaired. But drug testing is problematic when the goal is to increase worker productivity or maintain the public perception that a sport is fair. And it is quite a different matter if the goal is merely speculative or symbolic. In the case *National Treasury Employees Union* v. *von Raab* (816 F.2d 170, 1987), the Customs Service argued that drug use by Customs officials may lead to bribery or blackmail and that the integrity of the Customs Service needed to be maintained (Kamisar, 1987). In dissent, Justice Antonin Scalia wrote: "I think that this justification is unacceptable; that the impairment of individual liberties cannot be the means of making a point, that symbolism, even symbolism for so worthy a cause as the abolition of unlawful drugs, cannot validate an otherwise unreasonable search" (Kamisar, 1987, p. 177).

Second, the means of achieving the goal must be appropriate. Drug-testing programs must be scientifically sound, with proper confirmatory tests and adequate quality control. The confidentiality of test results and the privacy of those tested should be preserved to the greatest extent possible. If ethical duties or principles are overridden, we should still try to respect them as much as possible. These ethical concerns still carry validity and moral force, and we should try to preserve what we can of them (Beauchamp & Childress, 1983, p. 48). Thus, even if autonomy is overridden, we cannot dispense with respect for autonomy, liberty, and privacy. Test results should not be overinterpreted; even confirmed positive results do not necessarily indicate chronic drug abuse or impaired work performance.

Third, alternative means of achieving the goal should be considered or tried. To identify impaired workers, direct testing of job performance might be more effective. Similarly, to reduce drug use, such measures as education, counseling, and voluntary treatment programs are less intrusive. If they are shown to be ineffective, then drug testing of individuals would be more strongly justified.

Drug testing is not a goal to be pursued for its own sake. Rather, it is a means to achieve goals. Nor is drug testing alone sufficient to solve the problem of drug abuse. Identifying drug users should be only the first step in a comprehensive drug program. In addition to discussing drug-testing programs, the United States needs to develop effective counseling and rehabilitation programs and to make them available to drug users.

REFERENCES

Beauchamp, T.L., Childress, J.F. (1983). *Principles of biomedical ethics* (2nd ed). New York: Oxford University Press.

Bok, S. (1982). *Secrets.* New York: Pantheon Books, pp. 10–11.

Childress, J.F. (1982). *Who should decide? Paternalism in health care.* New York: Oxford University Press.

Cohn, L. (1987, December 31). How Walsh pushed 49er drug tests. *San Francisco Chronicle,* p. D1.

Council on Scientific Affairs. (1987). Issues in employee drug testing. *JAMA, 258,* 2089–2096.

Davis, K.H., Hawks, R.L., Blanke, R.V. (1988). Assessment of laboratory quality in urine drug testing. *JAMA, 260,* 1749–1754.

Engelhardt, H.T. (1986). *The foundations of bioethics.* New York: Oxford University Press.

Gaylin, W. (1987, April 24). On AIDS and moral duty. *The New York Times,* p. A 27.

Glantz, L.H. (1989). A nation of suspects: Drug testing and the fourth amendment. *American Journal of Public Health, 79,* 1427–1431.

Holden, C. (1987). Doctors square off on employee drug testing. *Science, 238,* 744–745.

Hoyt, D.W., Finnigan, R.E., Nee, T., Shults, T.F., Butler, T.J. (1987). Drug testing in the workplace—are methods legally defensible? *JAMA, 258,* 504–509.

Kamisar, Y. (1987, September 13). Drugs, AIDS and the threat to privacy. *The New York Times Magazine,* pp. 109–114.

Lo, B. (1988). Medical ethics. In W. Kelley (Ed.), *Textbook of internal medicine.* Philadelphia: J.B. Lippincott Company, pp. 3–5.

Miike, L. (1987, May 20). Testimony before House Committee on Post Office and Civil Service Subcommittee on Human Resources.

Polankoff, P.L. (1987, October). Commission's drug testing proposal "last resort" in controlling abuse. *Occupational Health and Safety,* 26–27.

President's Commission for the Study of Ethical Problems in Medicine and Biomedical and Behavioral Research (1982). *Making Health Care Decisions.* Washington, DC: U.S. Government Printing Office, pp. 41–51.

Thomas, K. (1989). Review of *A history of private life, Vol. III: Passions of the Renaissance,* Roger Chartier. *The New York Review of Books, 36,* pp. 15–19.

10

Drug Testing as Experienced by Mandatory Participants

ROBERT H. COOMBS

National concern about the widespread use of illegal drugs encouraged leaders in federal and local government, private industry, and professional athletics to implement drug-testing programs. The purpose is to identify drug users and effectively prevent them from further drug use.

Although the resulting controversy has been documented (Dougherty, 1987), and guidelines proposed (Pickett, 1986), little follow-up data is available and few outcome studies have been reported (Gust and Walsh, 1989). The popular press and the professional literature (Mallios, 1987; Rovere, Haupt, & Yates, 1986; Cowart, 1988a, 1988b) have highlighted the need for, and the problems associated with, drug testing, but only a few attitude surveys have been reported (Gaskins & deShazo, 1985; Abdenour, Miner, & Weir, 1987).

An opportunity to assess the personal impact of drug testing on those required to provide urine samples came when administrators of a major university (which shall remain anonymous) requested an evaluation of their mandatory testing program for intercollegiate athletes. Begun in 1986, this testing program was stimulated by media-focused concern about drug abuse among college and professional athletes and by the new policy of the National Collegiate Athletic Association (NCAA) to test athletes at national competitions for drugs. The objective was to protect the health and safety of all competitors, provide assistance for those identified as substance users, and prevent an unfair competitive edge by those who abuse certain chemical substances.

Each athlete was required to provide an initial urine sample during preseason medical evaluations. Substances tested included anabolic steroids, central nervous system stimulants, narcotic analgesics, psychomotor stimulants, and other drugs (PCP, marijuana, Quaaludes, barbiturates, and related substances). Those who tested positive were contacted by the team physician, offered voluntary counseling, and retested with randomly selected teammates. All students with positive first samples, plus several others selected on a random basis, were retested.

Positive results on the second test, confirmed with an immediate re-testing, resulted in mandatory counseling and notification of the head coach. Refusal to participate resulted in immediate suspension from all athletic participation, including practice sessions. Positive results on a third test brought about immediate suspension from all intercollegiate athletics and likely nonrenewal of an athletic grant-in-aid. A system to ensure due-process rights provided a hearing and an appeals process.

EVALUATION METHODS

Research means consisted of two data-collection methods: personal interviews and questionnaires. In 1987, interviews took place with 57 athletes obtained by random sampling from 624 student athletes. These interviews were tape-recorded and transcribed. Questionnaire data obtained from nearly all intercollegiate athletes supplemented this information. Privately completed during the initial team meeting at the beginning of the 1987–88 school year, these forms were confidentially submitted in sealed envelopes. No identifying information was revealed.

Five hundred drug-tested athletes were contrasted with a comparison group of 124 other intercollegiate athletes not required to give urine samples (mostly those on the crew teams). This comparison group was similar to drug-tested athletes in that they competed in intercollegiate athletics for the same university, were no different in marital status (about 97 percent of each group were unmarried), had the same expectations for graduation (99 percent of each group), and exhibited enthusiasm for their sport (about 56 percent of each group planned to participate in their sport after graduation).

Comparison subjects differed, however, in other ways: a smaller number were male (58 percent of the former and 71 percent of tested athletes), they were slightly younger (49 percent of the comparison group were freshmen compared to 33 percent of the tested students), and were less likely to have an athletic scholarship (6 percent as opposed to 31 percent, respectively).

This chapter highlights findings that address four research questions from participants' perspective: (1) How effective is mandatory drug testing in accurately identifying users? (2) How effective is drug testing in preventing drug use? (3) How does drug testing affect the personal lives of participants? And (4) How can the drug-testing experience be improved?

EFFECTIVENESS IN IDENTIFYING USERS

A considerable difference of opinion existed among athletes about the efficacy of urine testing in identifying users (Coombs & Ryan, 1990). Approximately two-thirds (68.7 percent) agreed and one-third (31.3 percent) disagreed with the questionnaire item, "Mandatory drug testing is effective in identifying athletes who use drugs." The high-technology equipment, "the most sophisticated in the world," was regarded by the majority of respondents as too precise and the monitoring system too rigorous to avoid detection. "With all your clothing stripped off and two guys watching you from five feet away," one respondent concluded, "it's next to impossible to cheat; there's no way you can alter the urine or use someone else's sample." Media accounts of athletes disqualified from competition because of positive test results reinforced this opinion. "It hits the front page of the sports section every time an athlete tests positive and is banned from playing," one individual remarked.

Knowledge of teammates who tested positive strengthened this view. A third (35.8 percent) of the tested athletes knew at least one drug-using athlete who had been caught (those in the comparison group were aware of significantly fewer). "The tests showed positive for a number of them," one observed. "They knew they were going to get caught. They were slapped on the wrist, encouraged to seek counseling, and randomly tested again about a month later." None were aware of anyone who had been more severely disciplined.

Drug testing, however, is not foolproof, as one-third of those responding pointed out. Despite high technology and rigorous monitoring, athletes knew effective ways to escape detection. Six of ten athletes (58.6 percent) disagree (23.6 percent strongly) with the questionnaire item, "There is no way to avoid detection when using drugs." Personal knowledge of drug-using athletes who had avoided detection reinforced this view. "I know guys who are heavy, heavy users that weren't caught," one acknowledged. "These guys do marijuana four or five times a week— almost every day—and they weren't caught."

"I know guys who did drugs four days before the test and weren't caught," another added. Asked how these false-negatives occur, one reflected, "I can't explain it; maybe drug testing is to make the athletic department look good and put people's minds to rest."

Athletes reported a variety of techniques to avoid detection, the most popular of which were: (1) the timing of drug use so substances clear the body before testing (stop-and-go technique), (2) the use of certain drinks, foods, or food supplements believed to dilute or disguise drug residue in the urine, and (3) the use of someone else's urine. Drug-tested athletes, compared to the comparison group, were significantly more knowledgeable about these techniques.

The first method, the stop-and-go technique, was most frequently mentioned. Twice as many tested athletes (40.3 percent, compared with 20.5 percent of the untested group) admitted being aware of detection avoidance via skillful timing of drug use ($p < .001$). When athletes anticipate a urine test, they simply avoid drugs long enough for the residue to clear the body. Educational sessions provided information about the length of time various drugs remain in the body and an underground network informally conveyed fairly accurate estimates of testing dates. "If you have an idea when the test is coming up, you lay off until it's over," one athlete explained, "then you begin again."

"Give or take a week or two," another added, "you can usually antic- ipate when the test will be given. You stop for a while so you will be clean for the test, then you can start up again."

An official notice alerted athletes that testing would occur during their preseason medical examination, so drug-using athletes stayed clean for the preceding month, then resumed their drug use until the next testing, usually for the NCAA finals. "You can usually count the days to do drugs," one admitted, "but if you're dumb enough to use them the day before, you'll get caught." Obviously the stop-and-go system is less ef- fective with unpredictable testing dates.

One-third (31.5%) of the tested athletes (and 14 percent of the compar- ison group, $p < .001$) considered the use of liquids and other substances effective in confusing the chemical analysis. Hearsay, rather than suc- cessful experiences, shaped these views. "I've heard that results can be masked by drinking this or that substance," one said. "I don't know if it's true, but people say that drinking a lot of water flushes out your sys- tem and dilutes the urine." Cranberry juice was also believed to be a good body cleanser. "It does something to the crystalline in the urine, or some- thing like that." Also mentioned were mineral water, castor oil, lemon juice, and other diuretics. Vinegar, the most frequently mentioned, re- portedly "screws up the test."

"Downing a glass of vinegar," however, "isn't worth the trouble," one commented. "I know players who tried it and threw up five minutes later."

"I can barely stand to smell it," another added. "It makes me nau- seous."

Vitamin pills and over-the-counter medications, some claimed, also confound the test results. Cold medications such as Contac or Sudafed, for example, reportedly obscure results by creating chemical reactions with the drugs. "Then you can tell them [the testers] that you're using these medications as decongestants for sinus problems."

The most extreme method mentioned purportedly involves excreting someone else's urine through a catheter. "The Russians have figured out how to do it," one athlete reported. "You have someone else's clean urine come through a tube from the bladder to your penis." He had no idea how this could be accomplished!

EFFECTIVENESS IN PREVENTING DRUG USE

Little consensus existed among participants about the preventative im- pact of drug testing (Coombs & Ryan, 1990). The majority regarded it as an effective deterrent; some thought it ineffective; a few perceived it as conducive to greater drug use.

Two-thirds (62.4 percent) of tested athletes agreed with the questionnaire statement, "Mandatory drug testing is an effective way to prevent drug use." Even more (76.0 percent) agreed that "Mandatory drug testing deters some athletes from substance use." More than twice as many drug-tested athletes (46.6 percent) as comparisons (21.5 percent) acknowledged that drug users worry about being identified. "It stopped me," one confessed. "I used to do marijuana and occasionally tried some other things, but since I've been here I only drink beer, and that's it."

Diminished drug use among teammates reinforced the belief that testing deters drug use. "I have a couple of friends who totally quit," one noted. "The team I play on is more drug free than before the program started. About five people have either quit or cut down due to drug testing. Most of them were lightweight users, borderline people who did it a few times, but now, with drug testing, they say, 'Forget it.'"

Fear that negative test results will jeopardize current and future opportunities motivated some to quit drugs. "Sports are up toward the top of the important things in my life and must not be jeopardized by drug-testing results," one athlete acknowledged. "I can't afford to mess up; I get 'paid' in lots of ways for my athletic skills. I come from a lower socio-economic background and athletics is my future!"

The deleterious effects that substances have upon bodies and minds caused less concern to most athletes than the possible loss of standing on the team. "People are much more worried about passing the test than about what the drug does to them," one respondent noted. "They now think twice before using the recreational stuff."

Team loyalty also acts as a deterrent. "The minute somebody gets busted," one explained, "it reflects on everybody. Drug testing has forced us to make a commitment to the team and has kept us clean."

Testing also provided a socially acceptable excuse for refusing drugs offered in friendship. "When my teammates and I are at a party and someone asks us if we want to get stoned—offers us a 'hit' off a 'joint,' or a 'piece of candy,' we say 'No, I can't, I'm going to be drug tested.' It gives us a way out."

The frequency of drug use among tested athletes, contrasted with those exempted (the comparison group), further assesses the preventative impact of drug testing. If testing exerts a preventative influence, significantly less drug use should be found among the tested athletes. The results show this to be true. Tested athletes used significantly less marijuana: one-third (30.8 percent) used this substance at least once during the testing year, compared to nearly half (46.2 percent) of the untested athletes ($p < .02$). Similarly, significantly fewer drug-tested athletes used other substances such as LSD, barbiturates, liquor, wine, and tobacco. This pattern was consistent for sixteen of eighteen substances.

As mentioned, not all athletes agreed that testing deters drug use. Only a third of interviewees who regarded testing as preventative gave an unqualified response; the remainder perceived it as only partially preventative and offered personal examples of ineffectiveness. Referring to the stop-and-go technique, one explained, "No drugs are taken before the test, but once in the clear we start up again; once it's over, life resumes."

In short, athletes can avoid detection by refraining from drug use for the length of time needed for various substances to clear the body. "Some drugs will be out of your system in a few days, while others will stay," one athlete explained. "You can usually figure out when the tests are going to be given and avoid being nailed. If you're stupid enough to take drugs before the testing date, you're an idiot."

A few athletes unabashedly continued their drug habits, preferring to take their chances and see what came. Because the testing system is not infallible and the first offense penalty is only a warning, there is little risk. "There's not much to lose the first time," one respondent explained. "It doesn't slow some guys down until they get caught the first time. They live-it-up until then and 'boom,' they lay off."

Results show that, despite drug testing, most drug-using athletes continued their former drug use pattern: 12.9 percent (62 athletes) smoked marijuana as often, 5.3 percent (25 athletes) used the same amount of cocaine, 3.6 percent (17 athletes) the same steroids, 64.0 percent (308 athletes) drank as much alcohol, 45.3 percent (217 athletes) used the same prescription drugs, and 57.5 percent (277 athletes) the same over-the-counter medications.

Surprisingly, some athletes actually increased their use of various substances: 2.3 percent (11) increased marijuana, 1.3 percent (6) increased cocaine, 0.6 percent (3) increased steroids, 9.2 percent (44) increased alcohol, 2.1 percent (10) increased prescription drugs, and 2.3 percent (11) over-the-counter drugs. These results are consistent with the questionnaire finding that one-sixth of the tested athletes (15.4 percent contrasted with 5.1 percent of the comparison group; $p < .01$) argued that drug testing encourages, not discourages, drug use. Citing themselves and their teammates as examples, these athletes slowed down temporarily; then after giving a urine sample, they increased their drug use. Before mandatory testing the use of recreational drugs was "no big deal." "They would do it every once in a while," one athlete explained. "But now, after being tested, they go right out and get stoned. 'Hooray! There won't be any more drug testing for a while.' People who normally wouldn't use drugs that much get together after testing and say, 'Let's celebrate.'"

However, except for use of alcoholic beverages, a larger proportion of tested athletes decreased their use of substances: 21.7 percent (104 athletes) smoked marijuana less often, 8.4 percent (40 athletes) used less cocaine, 2.5 percent (12 athletes) less steroids, 8.3% (40 athletes) less alcohol, 5.0 percent (24 athletes) fewer prescription drugs, and 8.1 percent (39 athletes) fewer over-the-counter medications.

Unexpectedly, the comparison subjects also reduced their drug use. Although not directly tested, the drug-testing milieu apparently influenced this group to decrease its drug use as well: 22.8 percent of the comparison group (26 athletes) used less marijuana, 2.7 percent (3 athletes) less cocaine, 1.8 percent (2 athletes) less steroid, 12.3 percent (14 athletes) less alcohol, 6.2 percent (7 athletes) fewer prescription drugs, and 5.3 percent (6 athletes) fewer over-the-counter preparations. The mandatory drug-testing policy apparently created a social climate that stimulated many athletes—both tested and comparison subjects—to reduce drug use. Yet the evidence shows that the drug patterns of most students remained the same, and a minority actually increased their use of substances.

IMPACT ON PERSONAL LIFE

Most drug-tested athletes were not disturbed by the testing experience; in fact, seven out of ten (71.4 percent) said that it had little or no impact upon their personal lives. "It was no big deal," the sentiment ran (Coombs & Coombs, 1990a, 1990b). "It took about fifteen minutes out of my year," one said. "After that I didn't give it another thought." "Most of us don't mind the drug testing," another added. "In fact, it sounded like a good idea. No one complained because we don't have a drug problem on our team."

Adverse Outcomes

Other athletes—a little more than a third (38.9 percent)—claimed that, though there were no lasting after-effects, the testing experience was stressful and their morale adversely affected. "I wasn't too happy about the whole thing," one complained. "It was a hassle."

Fear of being falsely identified as a drug user created anxieties. Nearly half (47.4 percent) worried about being inaccurately identified. "It scares me because I realize that, although the drug tests are basically very efficient, there may be a five percent chance of error. If I'm one of the five percent, it could ruin my reputation and my athletic opportunities."

Some athletes worried that the use of cold remedies and other over-the-counter medications might be mistaken for illicit drugs. Rumors circulated that some athletes had been disqualified from competition for using an asthma medication. "It isn't really fair to the athlete or his team to lose a big competition because someone takes a cold medicine," one argued.

Nearly half (47.2 percent) were chagrined by the testing experience. "It was embarrassing," one said, "but I knew that if I wanted to compete, I had to do it; so I just did it and got it over with."

"It was too impersonal," another added. "It was pretty embarrassing to be told, 'O.K., strip!' I lost a lot of respect for the athletic department."

Some participants described the testing experience as humiliating (36.8 percent) and upsetting (26.5 percent). The worst experience reported came from a young athlete tested at a national event. "My drug-testing experience at the nationals was very degrading, an invasion of my privacy," she said.

> Before the competition I thought I would be drug tested. 'Oh, no big deal.' But when they whisked me away right after the competition, I was very upset. They grabbed me and locked me into a room for three hours with a bunch of other athletes, gave me a gallon of water to drink, and said that I couldn't leave the room until I completed the drug testing. I was dehydrated, had stomach cramps and was very upset. I never got a chance to cool down and was very upset that I had to urinate in front of somebody I didn't even know. I felt that they were using me as a guinea pig; they didn't test people like this in other sports. I wasn't allowed to warm down, talk to my coach or teammates, or even receive my award—all the pleasant things that go with winning. I was very embarrassed and upset.

Beneficial Outcomes

Other athletes reported positive outcomes. More than a third (36.9 percent) viewed the testing as an interesting experience. Controversial and novel, with considerable media attention, drug testing provided participants with "a good story" to tell. Friends would remark, "Oh, you guys are getting drug tested? What's it like? We've heard a lot about drug testing in the pros and from college players banned from bowl games."

"It's an interesting conversation piece," one respondent reported. In such encounters, another noted, "Drugs now come up in conversation more as a negative than a positive."

One third (35.5 percent) of tested athletes described the experience as educational, as increasing their awareness of how drugs can damage the body (33.8 percent). "It has made me more aware of what I put into my body," one reported. "I realize that I have to be more careful."

The danger of secondary smoke from marijuana worried 15 percent of the interviewees. "I have to be a lot more careful about my social life," one stated. "If I'm in a room with people smoking marijuana, there is a possibility I might test positive. Being in the same room with people doing marijuana can give you 'contact buzz'." Finding themselves in such situations, these cautious athletes withdrew. "I had to leave my friend's room at a party and had to sit in the hall and talk to them through the door," one reported. "I had to stay away from the smoke so I wouldn't inhale and test positive."

Nearly a fourth of the tested athletes (23.3 percent) reported that drug testing has caused them to reduce their "partying." Some selected new friends. "I don't hang around with the people I used to because of what they do," one acknowledged. "When I'm around them when they smoke, I'm afraid I will breathe in [the smoke]."

"I'm a little more careful now about whom I party with," another respondent said.

"Before I go out with friends, I ask them what's on their agenda for the evening," still another reported. And, when drugs are offered, athletes now have a socially accepted excuse to decline. "It's easier now to say 'no'." More than half of all respondents (52.8 percent) credited the drug-testing policy as giving them a socially acceptable way to refuse drugs.

Some reported that their athletic performance and academic achievement also benefitted from drug testing. Slightly more than a quarter (27.0 percent) claimed improved athletic performance and 21.8 percent improved academic achievement.

IMPROVING THE DRUG-TESTING EXPERIENCE

Four of ten interviewed athletes (40.3 percent) could think of no improvement in the drug-testing system (Coombs & Coombs, 1990b). "They're going about it the right way," one concluded. "I'd adopt the same policy if I were in charge." However, others did propose improvements, which shall be discussed here.

Providing for Participant Dignity

The impersonal and insensitive way that urine samples were collected offended more than one-third of the male athletes, but none of the women. "That is my only problem with the whole thing," one male respondent said. Particularly bothersome was the underlying feeling of distrust that prevailed, the attitude that participants were guilty until proven innocent. "I felt that I wasn't being trusted, and it really bothered me," one athlete complained. "Maybe there are people out there who will cheat and pull tricks to pass the test, but I'm not one of them. It offended me!"

Feeling self-conscious and anxious, some male athletes were unable to urinate. "It's embarrassing to stand there for five minutes trying to urinate with three guys watching you to make sure you don't cheat," one complained. It didn't make things any easier when testers chided, "You stand there until you can go. You can't practice until you urinate into the bottle." One humiliated participant complained, "If you don't have to go, you can't go!"

Some unsuccessful participants reportedly had to come back three and four times: "Here I am stark naked trying to pee into a bottle," one complained. "It took me a while to relax. Finally, I was successful after going back four times and drinking a lot of water. It was pretty stressful going back and back."

Athletes recommend a setting that provides at least a modicum of privacy to maintain dignity, one that counteracts the implied feeling that they are cheaters. "It needs to be more sensitive and personal, less militant-like," was the consensus that was echoed.

Providing an Effective Educational Program

Many participants expressed (70.1 percent) the need for better drug education. Over half (52.9 percent) wanted more information about specific drug effects on the body. Information about the length of time that drugs remain in the body is valued, but most participants want more basic information, with fewer scare tactics.

To counteract the popularity and easy accessibility of drugs ("You can get them anywhere"), drug education must be understandable and persuasive to help at-risk individuals make informed decisions.

"When we were briefed on drugs and drug testing," one athlete reported, "it was too technical, too many long medical terms." Medical cataloguing of drugs and drug effects proved counterproductive for some. "I wish the doctors were more convincing," one said. "When I heard the presenters discussing the long- and short-term effects of drugs, I got the idea that it's okay to use them. The information helped me figure out how long before the test I needed to quit using."

Educational information presented by "uncool" doctors from an older generation was not taken seriously. "Guys who like to party consider drug education a joke, something stupid and useless. They sat there during the lecture looking at each other, thinking 'Ha, ha, ha.' Something more powerful is needed to reach them, such as big-name athletes who give personal examples of athletes whose lives have been ruined."

An effective instructional program, many asserted, must make clear that the intent is to help, not ruin, participants. An impersonal and militaristic approach conveys the opposite impression. This is how one athlete described his orientation: "'Here, read this and sign. If you don't sign, you can't play.' I skimmed it and signed because I wanted to play," he complained. "It would have been really helpful to have someone explain what I was signing, to make it clearer and help me interpret it. It would have reduced my anxieties and made me more comfortable." About half (49.5 percent) of tested athletes expressed a need for a better orientation as to what to expect.

Participants also emphasized the need for a comfortable educational and testing setting. Testing sites were reportedly too cold (57.8 percent) and crowded classroom settings too hot. "It's not easy to be enthusiastic or motivated by educational efforts when 110 big bodies have to sit compressed in a hot room," said one respondent.

More Reasonable Drug-Testing Objectives

One-fourth of interviewed participants (23.9 percent) criticized the list of tested drugs as too long. They acknowledged the appropriateness of testing for steroids and other performance-enhancing substances, but thought it "ridiculous" to test for other drugs. "I disagree with a list of thirty-five to forty substances," one athlete complained. "It's unfair when they're not performance-enhancing drugs."

"If the NCAA list continues to grow," another lamented, "pretty soon they'll be down to candy bars. Chocolate has caffeine."

"It's pointless to test for over-the-counter medicines like cough syrup," still another respondent complained. "Athletes don't take Anacin or Contac so they can play well. It's just too ticky-tacky. Mom made him take it and now he turns up positive and the whole team gets kicked out."

Athletes agree that it is appropriate to test for the following substances: steroids (92 percent agree); cocaine (88.8 percent), barbiturates (84.8 percent), heroin (87.7 percent), amphetamines (86.8 percent), tranquilizers (78.0 percent), marijuana (71.9 percent), tobacco (25.4 percent), prescription drugs (25.0 percent), and alcohol (24.5 percent). Tested athletes felt considerably stronger than do comparison subjects about testing for all these drugs except tobacco and prescription medications.

More Rigorous Drug-Testing Standards

Sixty percent of all tested athletes recommended that testing dates be less predictable (Coombs & Coombs, 1990b). "I know it would be expensive, but, if I were in charge, I'd spot-test people once a week. If you're going to do it at all, you might as well do it right," said one athlete. Randomized spot checking was recommended. "When I first came here, it was the *in* thing to get high on pot, but now cocaine is the *in* social drug—it's all over the place, at all the parties. We know it stays in your system about seven days at most, so if you know when the test is going to be given, you can clean up and it won't be detected. That's why a spot check would be better than predictable testing dates."

Elaborating on the stop-and-go technique, one athlete explained, "As it is now, drug testing is a joke. At the start of the season you know it's coming, so you can stay clean and pass the initial test. Every athlete I know has a way of finding out when the next test is coming up. I constantly hear people say, 'We're getting tested in six weeks. I can have it out of my system by then'."

Effective results can only be obtained when "everybody is tested every time," one athlete argued. "If you get a cross-sectional sample," he pointed out, "some of the guys who do drugs are not going to get caught. If you're going to help those who have drug problems, you need to catch them quickly and often so that they will realize that they need help. I know it would be expensive, but if the university is really concerned, that's the way to go about it."

Most athletes (78.5 percent) agree that drug counseling should be required for those testing positive the first time and that the system be tightened with stricter consequences. "They should let the coach know so that the player has to shape up. Some guys are hard-headed and will keep on partying unless things are tighter."

The policy is so lenient now, another observed, that "people get to thinking, 'If we are caught, it isn't any big deal. I can go right back to my sport.' A little stricter policy would open their eyes a bit and start them worrying about being out of their sport."

CONCLUSIONS AND RECOMMENDATIONS

These findings provide a rare, if limited, view of drug-testing program effectiveness. In some respects, the drug-testing program succeeded in meeting its objectives. All athletes learned what the university expected of them about illegal drug use, and many reduced their use of these substances, even some untested athletes. Moreover, the testing policy provided a ready excuse, a counterforce to peer pressure, to decline drugs offered in friendship and yet do it gracefully. However, despite threatening sanctions, some athletes still continued to use harmful substances. A few used more drugs after testing was implemented.

The following modifications would likely enhance testing objectives.

1. Implement less predictable testing dates. Though the ethics and legality of random testing are debatable, less predictable testing dates may counteract the "stop-and-go method" successfully employed by some athletes to avoid detection.

2. Replace the "criminal justice" attitude with an educational/therapeutic approach. Rather than catching "deviants," the manifest attitude should be one of helpful concern and education.

3. Provide ongoing in-service training for staff who collect urine samples or are involved in other ways. They should be taught how to conduct testing with minimal discomfort and to maximize the dignity of the participants.

4. Implement an effective educational program to orient participants about the purposes and benefits of drug testing, one that allows them to explore their personal feelings and the social factors that contribute to drug abuse. Rather than didactic presentations offered by authority figures from an older generation (which were largely ineffective, and sometimes counterproductive), educational sessions might consist of small discussion groups led by noted athletes or others talented in drawing out students in meaningful discussions about drugs and drug testing.

5. Address the problem of alcohol, the most widely used addictive drug, in educational sessions. Excluding this substance from drug testing sends an unintended message that alcohol is safe and acceptable. Many interviewed athletes are completely ignorant about the addictive and health-damaging effects of alcohol. Bombarded with advertisements, young athletes associate drinking with popularity, sex appeal, and enhanced athletic performance. "Beer is good for you," one respondent said. "Beer is good for carbohydrate loading the night before a sports performance," another added.

Some athletic teams exert considerable peer pressure on team members to drink. "At the beginning of the year, we had three team members who didn't drink," a senior boasted. "But now they do." Senior team members chided one athlete who stayed away from drinking parties. "If you want to be part of this team, you need to join us in our weekends."

6. Provide a systematic evaluation plan to assess the cost-benefit ratio of testing at regular intervals. Critical suggestions solicited from participants for improving testing conditions and circumstances will make athletes aware that their views are important and that their needs give direction to testing policy. An advisory committee of student athletes would contribute to this end.

REFERENCES

Abdenour, T.E., Miner, M.J., & Weir, N. (1987). Attitudes of intercollegiate football players toward drug testing. *Athletic Training, 22,* 199–201.

Coombs, R.H., & Coombs, C.J. (1990a, in press). The impact of drug testing on the morale of intercollegiate athletes. *International Journal of the Addictions. 26.*

Coombs, R.H., & Coombs, C.J. (1990b, in review). Intercollegiate athletes view of mandatory drug testing.

Coombs, R.H., & Ryan, F.J. (1990). Drug testing effectiveness in identifying and preventing drug use. *American Journal of Drug and Alcohol Abuse, 16,* 173–184.

Cowart, V.S. (1988a). Accord on drug testing, sanctions sought before 1992 Olympics in Europe. *JAMA, 260,* 3397–3398.

Cowart, V.S. (1988b). Random testing during training, competition may be only way to combat drugs in sports. *JAMA, 260,* 3556–3557.

Dougherty, R.J. (1987). Controversies regarding urine testing. *Journal of Substance Abuse Treatment,* 4, 115–117.

Gaskins, S.E., & deShazo, W.F. (1985). Attitudes toward drug abuse and screening for an intercollegiate athletic program. *Physician and Sports Medicine, 13,* 93–100.

Gust, S.W., & Walsh, J.M. (1989). *Drugs in the workplace: Research and evaluation data.* NIDA Research Monograph Series No. 91 (DHSS Publication No. ADM 89–16). Washington, DC: Alcohol, Drug Abuse and Mental Health Administration, U.S. Public Health Service, Department of Health and Human Services.

Mallios, H.C. (1987). Drug testing of student athletes: Storm clouds on the horizon. *Athletic Administration, 16,* 12–13.

Pickett, A.D. (1986). Drug testing: What are the rules? *Athletic Training, 21,* 331–336.

Rovere, G.D., Haupt, H.A., & Yates, C.S. (1986). Drug testing in a university athletic program: Protocol and implementation. *Physician and Sports Medicine, 14,* 69–76.

11

Identifying, Treating, and Counseling Drug Abusers

RONALD M. PAOLINO

When properly conducted and monitored through appropriate quality-assurance procedures, urine testing provides an objective and reliable tool for detecting drug use. Nonetheless, it must be remembered that regardless of the level of sophistication of the methodology employed, testing does but one thing—demonstrates the presence or absence of drug(s) in the urine. A number of questions need to be addressed once a confirmed positive urine has been obtained. For example, what is the source of the drug? Is it from the proper use of a prescribed or over-the-counter medication? Is it an aberrant result from something the individual ate or drank? For example, ingestion of poppy seed bagels may result in a urine positive for opiates. Is it the result of the misuse of prescribed medication or from the use of an illicit drug? How much drug is being used and what is the pattern of use? Are other drugs being used that were not detected by the test?

What should be done once a positive urine is found to be the result of inappropriate use or abuse of drugs? The consequences may range from not hiring an individual in a pre-employment situation, incarceration where drug use involves probation or parole violation, or treatment and rehabilitation. While rehabilitation may not be the appropriate option in all cases, one thing may be stated with certainty: Without rehabilitation one can only expect the abuser to continue using drugs. Despite its deterrent value, urine monitoring alone is not sufficient to maintain abstinence in the drug-troubled individual.

The success of a urine monitoring program within an organizational setting will be determined by the quality of the drug-testing policy that should be developed and put into place prior to the initiation of testing. Without a well-conceptualized policy, drug testing will, at minimum, be useless and, at maximum, produce serious problems for both the organization and those who are tested. Determining the meaning of a positive urine sample and deciding what should be done requires the evaluation and input of clinical personnel having both expertise and experience in the specialized field of drug abuse.

This chapter focuses on treatment and rehabilitation, and it is meant to serve as a background for understanding the problems of the drug abuser and the treatment available. Its purposes are to provide:

- A conceptual framework within which to view the phenomena of abuse and addiction
- A holistic, multifactor model of assessment and treatment formulation
- Insights and concepts gleaned over a fifteen-year period of providing direct drug treatment services to over 2,500 patients

WHO TAKES DRUGS AND WHY?

There is no picture of the "typical" drug abuser. The individual may be young or old, male or female, educated or uneducated, professional or nonprofessional, and from any socioeconomic class. Reasons for taking drugs are as varied as the number of users questioned. Drugs may be taken because of peer pressure. They may also be taken to "reward" the user for doing a good job or to commit suicide. Drugs are also taken to relieve boredom, anxiety, depression, panic, or stress; enhance self-esteem, efficiency, clarity of thought, self-awareness, sex, learning, appetite, religious experience, positive mood, or physical performance; decrease sexual drive, irritability, compulsion/craving, or anger. Successful treatment of the drug abuser requires a clear and concise understanding of these reasons and the factors that generated them.

It is a common misconception that only irresponsible, lazy, "bad," and criminally oriented individuals use, misuse, or abuse drugs. Unfortunately, this view often results in the "war on drugs" becoming a war on people, particularly in the workplace. In fact, one may find an abuser to be a conscientious, competitive, highly motivated and committed person who uses drugs to cope with personal and job-related stress. Throughout the years, the author has treated numerous individuals in this category, e.g., executives, pharmacists, nurses, and physicians. Factors contributing to abuse in such individuals include the following:

1. High-performance jobs with pressure to be consistently correct, efficient, creative, and productive.
2. Belief that they are too intelligent to become dependent or addicted. In this regard all addicts are alike; everyone believes that he or she is the exception who will not become addicted.
3. Affluence—having the money to pay for the drugs.
4. Belief, reinforced by society, that usual regulations and laws do not apply to them.
5. Easy access to drugs (physicians, nurses, pharmacists).

Because of their commitment to work and maintenance of high performance, impairment on the job is often one of the last symptoms seen in the impaired professional. By the time work is affected, the individual will probably already have experienced significant marital, family, financial, and legal problems. Whether professional or nonprofessional, once an abuser has become addicted, distinctions disappear with regard to the intensity of the craving and the extent to which the individual will go to obtain drugs.

IDENTIFYING CHARACTERISTICS OF THE DRUG ABUSER IN THE WORKPLACE

Within the workplace, the habitual abuser tends to exhibit a number of behaviors that comprise a characteristic profile. Abusers are more likely to be late for work with elaborate excuses for tardiness. There may be a change in the pattern of absenteeism with an increase in the incidence of extended absences. Requests for changes in work schedules are common along with increased difficulty in meeting deadlines and schedules. Requests for early dismissal or time off are higher than average, and there is an increase in work errors. Chances of an on-the-job accident are increased. Moreover, abusers are more likely to file a workers' compensation claim and to use greater than average amounts of sick benefits (NIAAA, 1984; Harwood et al., 1984).

The above performance changes are accompanied by personality changes. The abuser may exhibit a general increase in irritability along with mood swings. There may be a loss of memory for events or conversations along with confusion. Abusers tend to become more socially isolated and withdrawn—for example, eating lunch alone and avoiding co-workers. Increased complaints of physical pain and an enhanced interest in drugs may also be present.

A word of caution: Many of the symptoms/signs described above are also caused by work-related stress ("burnout") and poor organizational management style. Employers developing a drug-abuse program should consider stress management and management/leadership style assessment as an integral part of any comprehensive substance-abuse prevention and early intervention effort in the workplace.

NATURE AND CHARACTERISTICS OF DRUG ABUSE AND ADDICTION

Drug Misuse and Abuse

Drug abuse may be viewed as a continuum ranging from occasional to chronic, compulsive use. Although most people automatically think of illicit drugs when discussing abuse, statistics gathered by the Drug Abuse Warning Network (DAWN) concerning drug-related deaths and emergency room visits clearly indicate that drugs from legitimate sources are a major problem (Project DAWN, 1982). Drug misuse, the use of prescribed medications in a manner differing from that for which they were prescribed, appears to be a greater problem than are illicit drugs (American Medical Association, 1983). Drug abuse may be defined as the use of prescribed or illicit drugs contrary to social and legal mores for the express purpose of altering one's state of consciousness. Abuse is commonly associated with intoxication; impairment of physical performance, perceptions, social and occupational functioning; and legal problems. Continued use poses a hazard both to one's physical and mental well-being.

Addiction

The standard definition of addiction was originally derived from phenomena observed with the opiates. Repeated use of these drugs results in the development of tolerance necessitating the need for increased doses in order to obtain the desired euphoria or "high." Tolerance is accompanied by physical dependence in which abrupt cessation of the opiate leads to a withdrawal syndrome.

The absence of classical signs of physical dependence or dramatic physiological withdrawal effects initially led many experts to the erroneous conclusion that cocaine is not addicting. Subsequent data have unfortunately shown that, while not meeting the definition of addiction derived from the opiates, cocaine is indeed an extremely addictive agent. A new definition of addiction has been proposed, which is applicable to drugs other than the opiates (Smith, 1984). This definition includes the following three criteria:

- Loss of control in using the drug
- Craving and compulsion
- Continued use despite adverse consequences to self and others

It should be noted that this definition of addiction makes no reference to tolerance, physical dependence, withdrawal, or frequency of drug use.

A major difference between drug abuse and addiction is that abuse can usually be stopped at will, whereas addiction cannot. Not all abusers become addicts. Why some abusers progress to addiction is not known, although it has been estimated that 10 to 15 percent of the general population may be prone to do so. Progression of abuse to the stage of addiction is invariably accompanied by a decrease in judgment and deterioration of interpersonal relationships. The addict will often lie and steal from his own family in order to maintain his habit. Concerns about personal safety and health are lost. It is not uncommon for heroin addicts to use water from toilets to dissolve heroin before injecting it intravenously.

The American Medical Association (AMA) House of Delegates voted to consider drug dependencies as diseases. The AMA has for many years considered alcoholism as a disease. Whether in fact alcoholism is a "disease" in the medical sense of the word has yet to be proven. Nonetheless, conceptualizing it as such has resulted in a number of important consequences for the alcohol addict. First, it lifts the burden of guilt and shame from alcoholics so that they are more likely to seek treatment rather than see themselves as "weak-willed" individuals for being unable to break the bonds of addiction. Alcoholics who see the problem as not their fault are more likely to submit to treatment. A second important implication of the disease concept of alcoholism is that it has gotten the medical community involved.

Although there is no medical treatment for alcoholism at present, there has been a greater acceptance to treat the medical "consequences." Whether or not this will happen in the case of drug addiction remains to be seen. Anyone working in the field of addiction is aware of the general reluctance of physicians to get involved in the treatment of drug abusers. This is no doubt due, in part, to the lack of medical education in this field (Pokorny, Putnam, & Fryer, 1980). Another factor contributing to the reticence to treat drug abusers is the devalued image of the abuser as "manipulative," "sociopathic," and a "troublemaker." Unfortunately, this image is all too readily reinforced by the behavior of some addicts. Every physician has his or her favorite internship and residency stories of belligerent and boisterous drug users causing great commotion in the hospital emergency room in the middle of the night demanding drugs or requiring treatment for overdose. The fact of the matter is that this is not a representative view of the drug abuser.

Addiction is viewed as a chronic, life-long disease with periods of remission and relapse. As such, the notion of "cure" is inappropriate. Rather, the goal of treatment is to increase the length of periods of abstinence. In this regard, the concept of the process of "recovering" used with alcoholism should also be used when speaking of drug addiction. That is, an addict is to be considered as recovering rather than recovered regardless of the period of abstinence. The idea of addiction as a life-long condition with possible periods of relapse raises crucial questions regarding treatment, how one defines recovery, and anticipated performance in the workplace.

Addiction is a disease of denial. It is a disease that can be conceptualized as having the peculiar characteristic in which the cause (the drug) of the disease (addiction) produces a decrease in ability to recognize and accept what is causing the malady. Denial is employed not only by the addict but also by those close to the addict. For example, the addict's family and co-workers will often fail to recognize the problem despite the fact that they know of the individual's ingestion of drugs and the obvious presence of symptoms. The tendency is for all concerned to look for reasons other than addiction to explain the individual's behavior and problems.

With this in mind, it is crucial to emphasize that addicts typically do not seek treatment on their own. It is therefore imperative to assess carefully the reason behind an individual seeking treatment. The experienced substance-abuse treatment provider will not fall into the trap common among inexperienced health care providers attempting to treat addicts—taking the patient at face value. Health care workers such as physicians and nurses rely heavily on a patient's self-report of complaints and history, assuming the person to be a reliable historian without hidden or devious motives. The prevailing notion is that with the exception of patients seeking evidence for undisclosed medico-legal litigation or prescribed medications to maintain a drug habit, patients who seek treatment do so because they want to and they tell the truth. The treatment provider must be aware that this is *not* true for abusers and must carefully assess the role of primary and secondary gains. Secondary gains refer to nontherapeutic advantages the abuser hopes to attain by entering treatment without authentically engaging in it—for example, removing pressures brought by family and employer.

A MULTIFACTOR MODEL OF EVALUATION AND TREATMENT PLAN FORMULATION

Effective assessment, case conceptualization, and treatment plan formulation necessitate the use of a unifying model in which one collects, sorts, and organizes relevant data. Decisions as to how and which data to collect and what constitutes treatment and rehabilitation are determined by the treatment philosophy of the provider. This philosophy is the basis for the model that is consciously or unconsciously employed and is reflected in treatment. It is therefore imperative that clinicians have an explicit understanding of the cognitive and/or intuitive model guiding their thoughts and actions regarding the therapeutic enterprise. What is proposed here is the use of a multifactor interactive model that takes into account social, psychological/psychodynamic, biological, learning, and spiritual/existential aspects of human existence. It is based on a holistic view of what it means to treat a human being with a drug abuse problem rather than simply how to treat drug abuse.

Social Factors

Humans do not live in isolation. To be human means to be in community with others. Actions, encouragement, or discouragement by members of one's "community" (whether it be family, friends, or others) effects the individual's beliefs, self-concept, and behavior. Sharing and loving are central to a sense of well-being. When they are not present, one dies spiritually, mentally, and even physically. Drug abusers are enabled through misdirected caring. This enabling is fostered by the active process of denial by both abuser and "significant others." In this manner, abuser and significant others share a co-dependency on drugs. For these reasons, the evaluation and treatment processes must take into account the impact of significant others. Treatment plans should incorporate such individuals, keeping in mind that they may play powerful yet conflicting roles both as stressors and supports to rehabilitation and a healthy drug-free life. Examples of treatment modalities which focus on this factor are couples and family therapy. The notion of community support is also central to the self-help groups Narcotics Anonymous and Alcoholics Anonymous.

Psychological/Psychodynamic Factors

Treatment plans should incorporate information about the personality structure and mental status of the abuser. This includes assessment of affective states, level of intellectual functioning, and personality. Psychological testing should be done on each patient. Because drugs directly affect mental status, testing should be repeated after an individual has been drug free for several weeks. Psychodynamic factors (e.g., unresolved grief reaction) may play a role in continued drug abuse and must be considered. Many abusers have significant psychopathology for which drugs are sometimes used in an attempt to self-medicate. The specific drugs chosen often reflect the underlying psychopathology. For example, opiates may be selectively chosen to control rage, while stimulants such as cocaine may alleviate depression (Khantzian, 1974; Khantzian & Khantzian, 1984). Any treatment provider associated with a methadone maintenance program can relate stories of patients reporting the need for the drug just to feel "normal." These individuals are able to function well, maintain employment, and have positive interpersonal relationships as long as they are on methadone. Once detoxified there is a deterioration in adaptive functioning. While self-medication cannot be used to explain all drug-abuse behavior, it is a factor that must be carefully evaluated.

A positive relationship between chronicity of multiple drug addiction, including opiates, severity of psychopathology, and, specifically, personality disorders, has been found (Treece, 1984). It has been reported that 60 percent of young adult chronic psychiatric patients seen in a community mental health center were either actively using or had a history of using substances despite the fact that these individuals often denied illicit drug use (Safer, 1987). Substance abuse in these individuals exacerbated symptomatology, increased the rate of law violations, and resulted in 2½ times greater hospitalizations.

Biological Factors

The concept of self-medication has garnered support from the discoveries of opiate and benzodiazepine receptors in the brain (Snyder, 1978; Braestrup & Squires, 1978). Endorphins, considered to be naturally occurring opiate-like neurotransmitters, are found in the hypothalamus and limbic system, brain structures that play a key role in one's emotions. Studies have suggested these putative neurotransmitters are involved in depression, psychoses, and anxiety/panic disorders (Pickar et al., 1982). Thus, drug abuse in some individuals may result from attempting to compensate for deficiencies in naturally occurring endorphins.

Twin and adoption studies have led to the suggestion of a genetic link in the predisposition to alcoholism in the children of alcoholics (Goodwin, 1985). Future research may find a similar relationship for drug abuse. Unfortunately, a possible theoretical genetic link to abuse is, at this point, of little practical import to the treatment person sitting across from the drug abuser presenting for treatment.

A thorough medical examination including appropriate blood tests (liver function, hepatitis) should be part of the evaluation of the drug abuser. Many individuals seeking treatment are in dire need of medical attention for complications associated with drug abuse, such as hepatic disorders, bacterial endocarditis, and other septic conditions affecting the lungs and kidneys. Presenting psychiatric symptoms may also have their origin in medical disorders—for example, depression associated with abnormal thyroid functioning.

Learning Factors

Basic principles of learning theory apply to the phenomenon of drug abuse. It is a well-established fact that the probability of an elicited response is directly related to the procurement of reward or punishment. The closer in time between response and reward, the greater the chance of recurrence. Similarly, the greater the reward the stronger the connection between the stimulus and the response. It is also known that environmental cues present during the presentation of the reward acquire secondary reinforcing properties; the end result being that the probability of a conditioned response occurring is increased in the presence of these cues. This phenomenon can account for some IV drug users becoming addicted to the act of sticking themselves with needles. That is, pleasure is obtained from the injection even when no drug is used.

It has also been suggested that conditioned withdrawal responses may be elicited from environmental cues associated with actual withdrawal induced by the lack of drugs. This mechanism has been used to account for relapse in addicts who have been off drugs but who return to their old environment in which drugs were previously used (Wikler, 1948). Addicts also report what might be termed "conditioned anticipatory excitement" associated with drug-seeking behavior in which a sense of excitement and euphoria increases in intensity the closer the addict gets to obtaining and using drugs.

These examples demonstrate the powerful, learned conditioned responses associated with addiction. In addition to these simple forms of conditioning, one cannot overlook the more complex social learning that takes place—for example, when children observe parents using drugs for "recreational" purposes. In such instances children grow up with the message that it is all right to take drugs. Drug abuse may also result from attempts at compensating for poorly learned coping skills. Inadequately learned social skills or maladaptive thinking patterns may result in poor interpersonal relationships or a general lackadaisical state of existence from which the individual attempts to find relief through drugs.

Treatment modalities reflecting a learning theory approach include hypnosis, biofeedback, relaxation training, aversive conditioning, and cognitive restructuring therapy.

Spiritual/Existential Aspects

Anyone treating patients who have a drug problem is familiar with the frequent complaints of boredom, lack of meaning and purpose in life, and feelings of emptiness expressed by these individuals. They will often state that life is meaningless and without direction. A holistic assessment and treatment formulation must look at such complaints and assess their validity as true spiritual and existential issues to be addressed in treatment. Ignoring the spiritual and existential dimensions results in a simplistic, reductionistic view of the individual and his or her problems.

From an existential perspective, addiction decreases the freedom to choose from possibilities of existence open to the individual. Drugs, by producing overwhelming and powerful moods, limit modes of relating and responding to others. The use of drugs may thus be seen as an attempt to relinquish one's sense of responsibility to live authentically. Psychodynamic and learning theory schools of human behavior see humans from a deterministic point of view in which people are "pushed" into the future by their past. In contrast, from a spiritual/existential perspective people are seen as being "pulled" into the future by a sense of destiny and purpose.

Human beings are more than the summation of their past experiences. Each is his or her own unique potential projected into the future. In this sense, we are in a state of becoming what we can be. In this regard, it is interesting to note that many drug addicts have great difficulty in grasping the subjective sense of the future. When addicts are asked what they expect to be doing one month in the future, they will often respond with a look of bewilderment. This, of course, is an extremely important point since the rehabilitation process is predicated on the ability to set and work toward future goals.

Values, those principles constituting the unique and central image of self, provide meaning to life and guide behavior. They allow people to appreciate their unique existence and provide a consistent framework for relating to others. Dealing with the inevitable suffering in life is made possible by values. Facts become meaningful only when fitted within a value system, and values are reflected in behavior. Treatment should include an evaluation of the individual's value system—using and modifying it to serve as a structural framework within which the person may live a meaningful life in creative action and experience without drugs. Feelings and beliefs concerning issues related to guilt, choice, responsibility, forgiveness (of one's self and others), death, afterlife, sense of destiny, and God are all central to each individual human life. Spiritual and religious beliefs are at the core of a person's power to grow. However, at times these beliefs can be a source of anguish and maladaptation. These issues need to be assessed and incorporated into treatment where possible, not in a moralistic fashion but in a way that facilitates healing. At times direct spiritual counseling by clergy may be required. Narcotics Anonymous and Alcoholics Anonymous address both social and spiritual needs.

TREATMENT CONCEPTS AND COMPONENTS

What follows are principles and treatment modalities to be considered in the development of each treatment plan. Proponents of specific treatment approaches tend to overemphasize the importance of their approach over others. However, as mentioned elsewhere, abuse and addiction are complex phenomena and there is no single effective approach to rehabilitation. Each patient must be accepted as is and where he or she is at the time of entering treatment. The best approach is the one that works for a given individual.

Total Abstinence

This principle applies to all cases of drug abuse. However, this is not always possible, as in the cases in which narcotics are needed for chronic pain management and yet are abused by the patient. Otherwise, the notion of controlled substance use in the abuser is inappropriate and total abstinence must be sought. Drug-abuse treatment begins only after abstinence has been achieved.

Abstinence from Other Psychoactive Drugs

Generally speaking, the use of any psychoactive drug by the addict increases the chance of relapse. It is therefore important to eliminate the use of such medications. Once again, this is not always possible; for example, with severely depressed or anxious patients. With respect to cocaine use, often a clear correlation exists between the use of cocaine and alcohol. Even small quantities of alcohol may result in the relapse of the cocaine abuser who has been off drugs.

Education

Education is an essential part of the drug rehabilitation process. Individuals need to learn about the detrimental effects of drugs on physical and mental health, relationships with others, etc. Treatment modalities under this heading include social skills training, cognitive restructuring, psychoeducational groups, stress management, and biofeedback.

Family Involvement

Substance abuse affects the entire family and not just the abuser. Family members become co-dependent. Treatment must therefore involve family members if it is to be truly effective.

Individual/Group Psychotherapy

Individual psychotherapy is useful in providing patients with insight as to how and why drugs have become a significant part of their lives. One also learns what needs to be changed and how to bring about such changes. Group therapy provides the dimensions of community and learning through peers within a structured social therapeutic context.

Contingency Contracting

A controversial approach, contingency contracting works well with individuals who are highly motivated to stop using drugs. It appears to be particularly successful with professionals such as lawyers, nurses, pharmacists, and physicians who wish to put the drug problem behind them and get back to the practice of their profession. A contract is formulated and agreed upon by the patient stating that, in the event of relapse, the treatment provider is authorized to contact the individual's supervisor, professional review board, or governing body. The stakes are high with this approach since it may in fact mean a loss of professional license or ability to practice.

Alternative Activities

Drug abusers often lose the ability to enjoy ordinary pleasurable events or activities of everyday life. Cocaine abusers in particular report this, stating that all other pleasures pale in comparison to the cocaine "high." Consequently, learning or relearning to enjoy and getting involved with constructive, satisfying activities and hobbies are often an essential part of the drug rehabilitation process.

Self-Help Support Groups

The most common self-help groups are Narcotics Anonymous (NA) and Alcoholics Anonymous (AA). Based on the principle of total abstinence, NA and AA are independent nonprofit organizations. Membership consists of "recovering" addicts whose interest is to assist themselves and others in achieving and maintaining abstinence from drugs on a day-at-a-time basis. Both organizations are founded on twelve steps or principles related to spiritual awakening. Similar groups are available for the addict's co-dependents; for instance, Nar-Anon and Al-Anon for adults and Al-Ateen for youngsters. Participation in psychotherapy conducted by mental health professionals and involvement in either NA or AA are not mutually exclusive and, in fact, it is wise to advise concomitant involvement.

Therapeutic Communities

Therapeutic communities are self-help communities based on the notion that substance abusers are able to help themselves and each other. The goal is extensive restructuring of the abuser's life, personal goals, and priorities. It is believed that this is best achieved through the vigorous confrontation of the addict's drug-abusing mode of existence and thinking. As might be expected, this approach seems to work better with the more "entrenched" antisocial type of addict rather than individuals in early stages of addiction or those who are of a more psychologically fragile nature. Because of the expected long length of stay (six months to two years), external motivation such as court referral is usually necessary to ensure that participants remain with the program.

Half-Way Houses

Half-way houses are transition facilities for individuals who have been hospitalized. They are a rehabilitation option between hospitalization and living independently. Self-help oriented, they are oftentimes based on the philosophy of NA and AA. The expected length of stay in a half-way house may be two months to one year.

TREATMENT PLANS

Individualized treatment plans are developed utilizing information collected during an initial assessment phase.

Treatment goals should be stated in measurable terms so that therapeutic progress may be accurately evaluated. Goals need to be identified, developed, and given priority with input from the patient. A behaviorally oriented approach to treatment plan formulation is useful. Basic elements of such a system are as follows.

Problems—Specific, concisely defined problems to be resolved in treatment are agreed upon by both counselor and patient.

Goals—Goals for resolving stated problems are operationally defined.

Plans—Specific steps are listed in order to accomplish said goals.

End points—Criteria are clearly stated by which both patient and counselor know when a particular goal is achieved.

Logical consequences—Statement of logical consequences to occur if the goal is not attained. This step will be self-evident when the other elements are well thought out and optimal treatment has been provided.

Review—The final treatment plan is reviewed and signed by both patient and counselor.

INPATIENT VERSUS OUTPATIENT TREATMENT

One of the first questions to consider in treatment is whether the patient should be placed in an inpatient rehabilitation program or treated on an outpatient basis. There is no compelling evidence to warrant the belief that inpatient treatment should automatically be chosen. Drug-abuse treatment is still in its early stages of development and there are not sufficient data to compare the efficacy of inpatient versus outpatient treatment. There is, however, a significant amount of information regarding alcohol treatment, and the generally held view of the superiority of inpatient treatment has been questioned (Holden, 1987). With the exception of instances of life-threatening withdrawal syndromes (e.g., from barbiturates), there is no a priori reason automatically to choose inpatient drug-abuse treatment. Most treatment can be done on an outpatient basis. There are, however, circumstances that do warrant choosing inpatient over outpatient treatment. These include:

1. Loss of control in using drugs/alcohol
2. Serious health problems requiring inpatient medical attention
3. Psychiatric disorders requiring inpatient treatment
4. Social isolation or withdrawal
5. Absence of social/family support
6. History of repeated failure with outpatient treatment
7. Severe immediate consequences of relapse (loss of job, incarceration)

Once it has been decided that an individual needs inpatient treatment, an appropriate program must be chosen. Clearly, not all programs are equal in quality, and certification does not guarantee quality of care. A number of criteria are useful in making the choice.

1. Referral source's past experience with a program. History of program effectiveness as known by the referral source is probably the most pragmatic criterion
2. Ability to provide treatment components listed elsewhere in this chapter
3. Availability of medical back-up
4. Effectiveness of working relationship with NA and AA
5. Ability to treat dual diagnoses (e.g., addiction and psychiatric disorder)
6. Ability to provide effective follow-up plan
7. Ability to monitor treatment progress effectively
8. Willingness to interface with the referral source

PRINCIPLES RELATING TO TREATMENT

• *Substance abuse must be treated holistically.*

One does not treat a specific drug problem but a whole human being who has, among other things, a drug problem. Drug abuse permeates the individual's entire existence and mode of relating to others. Substance abusers often have serious difficulties in many aspects of their lives (i.e., marital, financial, interpersonal, medical, psychological, spiritual, and legal). Effective treatment/rehabilitation must assess and address the individual's entire life situation.

• *Substance abusers usually use multiple drugs, including alcohol.*

Polydrug abuse is the rule rather than the exception. Successful polydrug abuse treatment is both complex and difficult. Often the drugs abused are prescribed for medical or psychiatric reasons. This factor complicates matters.

• *Substance abuse affects not only abusers but also others.*

While data are not available for drug abuse, it is estimated that for every alcoholic as many as six to seven additional people (family and co-workers) are also affected (NIAAA, 1984). Thus, there is no reason to believe that this is not true also for drug abuse. Successful treatment must involve family members.

• *There is no specific treatment for specific drugs.*

Aside from specific medical or pharmacological considerations (e.g., barbiturate detoxification) treatment efforts need to be directed to the abuser and not the drug. Certain abusers (e.g., those who use cocaine) consider themselves special because of the drug they use. In the past this may have been true to some extent. However, because of increased drug availability and purity along with decreased price, differences in socioeconomic, educational, and employment factors between users has decreased dramatically. While differences exist between individual drug users, these differences should not automatically be attributed to the drug abused.

- *Effective substance abuse treatment requires a thorough psychological, social, and medical assessment.*

Successful holistic treatment is predicated on the assumption that a complete evaluation of the abuser has been made in a systematic and orderly fashion. A significant number of substance abusers have psychological problems that either preceded drug use or resulted from use. If the problems predated use, the individual may be using drugs as an attempt to self-medicate.

- *Substance abusers do not seek treatment voluntarily without some external pressure.*

This is particularly true when abuse has proceeded to the chronic state of addiction. It must be remembered that addiction is a disease of denial characterized by loss of control. As such, one does not expect addicts to admit to themselves or others that they have a problem. Consequently, "coercion" or pressure is generally necessary for addicts to enter treatment. Whenever an addict appears to be requesting treatment on his or her own, the treatment provider can rest assured that there is some external motivation. Common external motivators include threats of divorce or separation from one's spouse or children, fear of impending court action, and concern about losing one's job. The treatment provider should not be discouraged by this fact, but rather should utilize the opportunity at hand to begin treatment with no false illusions or naive optimism about the difficult task ahead. Unfortunately, some individuals seek treatment simply to reduce their level of tolerance to drugs in order to decrease the amount of money needed to maintain a desired habit.

- *Because of the nature of the professional training received by physicians, nurses, and other health care providers they tend to be easy "targets" for manipulation by addicts.*

Health care providers are motivated by a desire to help the afflicted and a need to nurture. They are "givers." Physicians and nurses in particular are accustomed to patients openly asking for help and complying with prescribed treatment. Individuals caught in the grip of addiction do not fit this mold. The overriding compulsion is to continue taking drugs through deviousness, deception, and manipulation if called for. The mode of existence of the addict is "taking" rather than giving.

- *Once in treatment, the addict will often attempt to develop an alliance with the treatment provider for the express purpose of removing the external pressure that forced him or her into treatment.*

This is usually seen during initial stages of treatment in which the addict's interest in rehabilitation is often minimal. Addicts tend to perceive themselves in treatment only because they have been forced to be there (which is often the case). Compliance may appear to be good until requests for letters to employees, judges, spouses, parole officers, etc., are denied, at which time the person may abruptly leave treatment.

- *Treatment efforts and decisions are often "contaminated" by the counselor's fear of the addict.*

Regardless of whether or not the treatment provider is experienced, there is always a certain degree of fear associated with treating addicts. This may not be an overt fright, but rather a more subtle state of anxiety (reinforced by fantasy) about what the addict might do if he or she does not get his or her way. Inexperienced counselors may not be aware of this fact. An experienced counselor knows that consciously or unconsciously there is always an element of intimidation related to treating addicts. The problem with not realizing this is that the counselor may unknowingly structure the situation so that the abuser either leaves treatment on his own or is terminated for not adhering to treatment guidelines. This is particularly true in treatment programs where program guidelines may be unconsciously manipulated by staff in order to exclude patients who do not fit the unwritten standards of the "ideal" patient. A knowledgeable counselor or treatment team recognizes the presence of this dynamic and establishes quality-control measures to ensure that it does not negatively influence the quality of care.

"Streetwise" abusers are very much aware of this dynamic and oftentimes attempt to exploit it with speech and subtle or not so subtle behaviors that may be interpreted as threatening or hostile. A healthy concern for the often impulsive and hostile nature of the addict, particularly when the person is actively using drugs, is necessary. However, the counselor needs assistance when this concern gets to the point that it affects the quality of care.

- *Addicts have an ability to "split" members of a treatment team.*

Abusers have an uncanny ability to be "emotional chameleons," changing their mode of emotional and behavioral presentation to match the needs of the moment. This selective presentation is particularly evident with the sociopathic personality but is a common aspect of the manipulative style of the abuser in general. Within treatment program settings where there is more than one individual involved in the abuser's treatment, this may lead to a "splitting" of staff in which members find themselves in conflict over various aspects of the patient's care. Treatment team members must be sophisticated enough to recognize this divisive action and function in a cooperative, integrated fashion.

- *Treatment must include firm setting of limits.*

Drug abusers constantly test limits with the counselor. This will take a variety of forms depending on the skill of the abuser and the weaknesses and strengths of the counselor as perceived by the abuser. One reason abusers do this is to get their own way. Another is that they may be testing the counselor's competence as he or she struggles with the conflict of committing oneself further to treatment. Abusers often perceive the counselor as their "last hope" to change their lifestyle. This hope is resisted because of an impaired ability to trust others. By understanding this process, the counselor avoids personalizing the abuser's attempts and proceeds with treatment in a caring but firm way.

CHARACTERISTICS OF AN EFFECTIVE COUNSELOR

• *An effective counselor is both caring and knowledgeable.*

Effective counselors are those who are knowledgeable about various techniques and treatment modalities. They must also be self-confident and flexible in their approach, using whatever "technique" is appropriate at a given point in time rather than trying to employ the same technique on every patient.

The second important characteristic is that of caring. Counselors may have a vast amount of technical knowledge but not possess a true concern for the welfare of the abuser. If this is the case, the person will not be effective since knowledge without caring is sterile. The counselor will not "connect" with the patient. Care without knowledge, on the other hand, is sentimental and ineffective.

• *An effective counselor is nonjudgmental.*

Each counselor has a personal value system that will be reflected in the individual's behavior and demeanor. However, moralizing or lecturing the abuser serves no useful purpose. The abuser has been lectured and been made to feel guilty by many others prior to entering treatment without any beneficial effect. Thus, counselors must be aware of their own attitudes about substance abuse and make every effort to ensure that negative attitudes do not hinder the rehabilitation process.

The function of the counselor is to counsel. Counselors have no moral or existential authority over patients, and there is no a priori reason to believe that patients will behave, think, or feel the way counselors expect them to. In fact, a patient may respond contrary to the counselor's suggestions in order to test the limits of the therapeutic relationship and the counselor's competence, particularly in early stages of treatment. This calls for a clear understanding of the counselor's purpose and limitations. The patient is free to follow or reject the counselor's recommendations.

• *An effective counselor does not enable the abuser.*

While abusers are free to choose and make decisions, they are also responsible for these choices. It is the counselor's role to make the individual aware of these responsibilities and to initiate logical consequences. In this regard the counselor differs from "significant others" who, through misguided caring, perpetuate the individual's maladaptive thinking and behavior. While sympathy is an essential part of caring, being overly sympathetic results in a counselor becoming "de-skilled." The end result is an enabling of the abuser and of the abuser's problems.

- *An effective counselor does not allow the individual to delay confronting the drug-abuse problem.*

Among the myriad of excuses used by abusers to avoid facing their problem is the belief that things will get better with time. They won't. Things can and will get worse if abuse has proceeded to addiction. The counselor must let the abuser know this. As part of rehabilitation, abusers must be made aware of inconsistencies in their thoughts, feelings, and behavior. This is done in a caring and sensitive manner so as to facilitate the therapeutic process.

ROLE OF URINE TESTING

Drug abusers are caught in a web of deceit and lies. It is not realistic to expect them to come forward on their own to ask for treatment. Most abusers enter treatment reluctantly as the result of a crisis—that is, having been given an ultimatum by loved ones or those in authority. Even then, the abuser tends to deny the extent of the drug problem. Excuses given by drug abusers to cover up or explain away their drug problems are creative and limitless. In a word, one cannot believe the abuser and, particularly, the addict who is in the active stage of using drugs. Patients will lie as to which drugs they are using as well as to how much is being used. This is the nature of the disease. For this reason, urine testing is an invaluable tool in the detection and early intervention of drug abuse as well as in the rehabilitation and follow-up processes. Testing provides an accurate method of determining which drugs are being used. Once an abuser is in treatment, urinalysis provides an objective and impartial method of confirming abstinence. When the patient completes treatment, testing serves as an effective deterrent to relapse and should be continued for six months to one year as part of the follow-up plan. Urine testing is an essential component of effective outpatient treatment.

QUALITY ASSURANCE PROGRAMS
FOR TREATMENT

While the need for quality assurance (QA) programs in drug testing is an accepted fact, this concept has yet to be applied to the field of drug-abuse treatment and rehabilitation. Patients, families, employers, and insurance companies underwriting drug treatment are plagued with questions related to the clinical and cost-effectiveness of specific treatment providers and programs. One often hears the argument that the process and outcome of rehabilitation do not readily lend themselves to measurement and evaluation. Regardless of theoretical orientation, any well-conceived and formulated treatment program and individualized treatment plan can be objectively evaluated and monitored. All drug programs appear great on paper or in radio/TV promotions written by their public relations departments. Invariably, these programs are expensive. Choosing among outpatient, inpatient, or residential treatment providers is a difficult task, as is evaluation of the effectiveness of treatment. However, evaluation of treatment effectiveness can and should be done. Employers contracting for drug-treatment services should insist on the option of unannounced audits conducted by independent qualified clinical personnel.

REFERENCES

American Medical Association. (1983). *Informal Steering Committee on Prescription Drug Abuse: Prescription Abuse Data Synthesis (PADS), data integration, and analysis model.* Working draft.

Braestrup, C., & Squires, R.F. (1978). Brain-specific benzodiazepine receptors. *British Journal of Psychiatry, 133,*249–260.

Goodwin, D.W. (1985). Alcoholism and genetics: The sins of the fathers. *Archives of General Psychiatry, 42,*171–178.

Harwood, H., Napolitano, D.M., Kristiansen, P.L., & Collins, J.J. (1984). *Economic costs to society of alcohol and drug abuse and mental illness: 1980.* Research Triangle Park, NC: Research Triangle Institute.

Holden, C. (1987). Is alcoholism treatment effective? *Science, 237,*20–22.

Khantzian, E.J. (1974). Opiate addiction: A critique of theory and some implications for treatment. *American Journal of Psychotherapy, 28,*59–70.

Khantzian, E.J., & Khantzian, N.J. (1984). Cocaine addiction: Is there a psychological predisposition? *Psychiatry Annals, 14,*753–759.

National Institute of Alcohol Abuse and Alcoholism (NIAAA). (1984). Fifth Special Report to the U.S. Congress on Alcohol and Health from the Secretary of Health and Human Services (DHHS Publication No. ADM 84–1291). Washington, DC: U.S. Government Printing Office.

Pickar, D., Extein, I., Gold, P., et al. (1982). Endorphins and affective illness. In N.S. Smith & A.G. Donald (Eds.), *Endorphins and opiate antagonists in psychiatric research: Clinical implications.* New York: Plenum Press.

Pokorny, A., Putnam, P., & Fryer, J.E. (1980). Drug abuse and alcoholism teaching in U.S. medical and osteopathic schools, 1975–1977. In M. Galanter (Ed.), *Alcohol and drug abuse in medical education.* Rockville, MD: National Institute on Drug Abuse.

Project DAWN (Drug Abuse Warning Network). (1982). Annual Report, 1981. Rockville, MD: National Institute on Drug Abuse.

Safer, D.J. (1987). Substance abuse by young adult chronic patients. *Hospital and Community Psychiatry, 38,*511–514.

Smith, D.E. (1984). Diagnostic, treatment and after-care approaches to cocaine abuse. *Journal of Substance Abuse Treatment, 1*,5–9.
Snyder, S.H. (1978). The opiate receptor and morphine-like peptides in the brain. *American Journal of Psychiatry, 135*,645–652.
Treece, C. (1984). Assessment of ego function in studies of narcotic addiction. In L. Bellack & L.A. Goldsmith (Eds.), *The broad scope of ego function assessment.* New York: John Wiley & Sons.
Wikler, A. (1948). Recent progress in research on the neurophysiological basis of morphine addiction. *American Journal of Psychiatry, 105*,329–338.

Index

Absenteeism, due to substance abuse, 166, 183
Absorption, of drugs in body, 51
Abstinence, total, 224
Abusers, drug
  attitudes toward, 219
  characteristics of, 216–17
  evaluation of, 222
  identification of, 203–5, 217
  nature of, 217–18
  "streetwise," 230
Accuracy, issue of, 88, 164–66
Accidents
  alcohol related, 18–19
  Conrail, 40
  related to drug abuse, 183
  U.S.S. *Nimitz*, 23, 94, 107
Addiction
  definition, 218
  nature, 53, 218–20
Adler, Allan, 34
AIDS, 136
Air Force, U.S. *See also* Military
  implementation of drug testing in, 99
  laboratories available to, 100
Air Force Special Action Program, 95
Al-Anon, 226
Al-Ateen, 226
Alcohol
  abuse, 5
  adverse effects of, 5
  athlete use of, 129–31, 207
  and cocaine use, 55, 224
  early screening programs for, 8
Alcohol, Drug Abuse and Mental Health Administration, 196
Alcohol abuse, costs of, 15, 18–19
Alcoholics Anonymous, 7, 221
Alcoholism
  concept of, 219
  genetic predisposition to, 222
Alcohol Rehabilitation Centers (ARCs), of U.S. Navy, 107, 108
Alprazolam (Xanax), 57, 58
Amalgamated Transit Workers Union, 28

Amateur sports, drug testing in, 13–15, 135. *See also* Athletics; Sports
American Academy of Occupational Medicine, 32
American Academy of Psychoanalysis, 32
American Association of Bioanalysts, 80
American Association for Clinical Chemistry (AACC), 80
American Bar Association (ABA), 39
American Civil Liberties Union (ACLU), 25, 31, 34, 36, 183, 185n
American Council on Education, 137
American Federation of Government Employees, 34
American Medical Association (AMA), 18, 20, 219
American Occupational Medical Association (AOMA), 31, 38
American Society for Promotion of Temperance, 5
Amobarbital, 64
Amoco, 39
Amphetamines
  banned by IOC, 15, 117
  interpretation of test results for, 87–88
  used by athletes, 129, 130
Anabolic steroids, 113
  action of, 116–17
  banned by IOC, 14
  efficacy of, 125
  masking of, 125–26
  problem of, 123–28
  research on, 124
  side effects associated with, 120–21
  testing for, 13–14, 127–28, 134
Analgesics, banned by IOC, 14
Anti-anxiety drugs, 57–58
Anti-Drug Abuse Act (1986), 33
Anxiolytics, 57
Arbitration cases, labor, 172
Arbitrators, role of, 162–63, 167
Armed Forces Institute of Pathology (AFIP), 102
Army, U.S. *See also* Military
  implementation of drug testing in, 99

235